Practical and Professional Ethics

VOLUME THREE
Biomedical Ethics

Practical and Professional Ethics Series

Vol. 1: The Primer of Applied Ethics
Vol. 2: Environmental Ethics
Vol. 3: Bio-Medical Ethics
Vol. 4: Educational Ethics
Vol. 5: Economic and Business Ethics
Vol. 6: Socio-Political Ethics

About the Author

Mr. Debashis Guha, teaches Ethics and Phenomenology and Existentialism in the Post Graduate Department of Philosophy, Ranchi University, Ranchi. After doing masters course in Philosophy from Delhi University in 1980, he was conferred the Ph.D. degree of Jadavpur University in 1988. Dr. Guha takes interest in Philosophy of Religion, Social and Political Philosophy, Philosophy of Science and Analytic Philosophy. He taught at the undergraduate level in a constituent college of Ranchi University from 1981 to 1989 and was then asked to serve the Post Graduate Department. Dr. Guha is teaching Ethics for twenty-four years. He was awarded the Visiting Associateship of the U.G.C. (1994-96) in Jadavpur University, Calcutta, where he worked out *An Inquiry into the cases of Pain and Suffering,* which awaits publication. He was further awarded U.G.C.'s Major Research Project (1997-2000) on *Applied Ethics in Indian Context,* which has been now shaped in Six volumes, of which the present work is the third one under the series: **Practical and Professional Ethics**. Dr. Guha has fourteen papers to his credit. He has presented philosophical papers in different Seminars, Symposia and Congress, two of them were presented in International Congress; one in the Platinum Jubilee Celebrations of the Indian Philosophical Congress, 2000-01, and the other in the XVth International Congress of Aesthetics in Tokyo, Japan in 2001. During his Major Research Project work, Dr. Guha has talked to many people from different walks of life, interviewed them and also arranged ethical dialogues leading to resolution of value-laden practical problems of urgency. Dr. Guha envisions peoples' participation in Practical and Professional Ethics.

Practical and Professional Ethics

Volume-Three

Biomedical Ethics

DEBASHIS GUHA

CONCEPT PUBLISHING COMPANY, NEW DELHI-110059

Cataloging in Publication Data—DK
Courtesy: D.K. Agencies (P) Ltd. <docinfo@dkagencies.com>

Guha, Debashis.
Practical and professional ethics / Debashis Guha.
v. 3 cm.
Includes bibliographical references.
Includes index.
Contents: v. 3. Biomedical ethics.
ISBN 8180693147 (set)
ISBN 8180693678 (v. 3)

1. Applied ethics. 2. Professional ethics. 3. Environmental ethics. 4. Bioethics. 5. Medical ethics.
I. Title.

DDC 170 22

ISBN 81-8069-314-7 (Series)
ISBN 81-8069-367-8 (HB)
ISBN 81-8069-368-6 (PB)

First Published 2007

Published and Printed by
Ashok Kumar Mittal
Concept Publishing Company
A/15-16, Commercial Block, Mohan Garden
New Delhi-110059 (INDIA)

Phones : 25351460, 25351794
Fax : 091-11-25357103
Email : publishing@conceptpub.com

Rishita

and

Reeju

Foreword

About 6 million years ago somewhere in Africa a species of apes *Homo sapiens* (meaning: man the wise) differentiated itself during the long process of evolution from rest of its counterparts. It could walk erect on its two posterior limbs or legs while two anterior limbs became hands. This species was also mentally highly evolved for it had acumen to think, decide and act wisely. It could communicate among its individual members with the help of signs, signals, sounds and gestures which later developed into some kind of primitive language. With the discovery of fire he marched forward on the road to modern civilization and captured the earth developing many languages, cultures, philosophy of life, discoveries and inventions. All these led to the development of a sustainable social order which was bound by economy, justice and ethics. At the present moment man is ecologically the most successful species on this planet.

Higher ideal of biological and social well-being of man's moral crisis in many issues in biology and medicine forms an important part in ethical discussions these days. This has become more important in the today's globalized world where everything is being decided by the market forces in accordance with the guidelines of the World Trade Organisation (WTO). During writing of the book "Biomedical Ethics", which is the third volume of the Series: "Practical and Professional Ethics" Dr. Debashis Guha has disturbed, interrupted, interrogated, discussed, e-mailed and corresponds with a great variety of people on the subject matter of this book. In this book he has discussed several value-laden issues of public health care including biological materials, namely human organs, tissues, cells, genome, genes and gene products as well as human cloning. Although an interesting and intricate subject in philosophy. Biomedical Ethics is of considerable importance for the social well-being of man and the human society. We should hence strengthen the teaching of biomedical ethics in our universities. This book is hence a timely contribution.

25/6/06

Narsinha Dayal
Plant Breeder & Cytogeneticist
Former Professor & head,
Department of Botany
and
Dean, Faculty of Science,
Ranchi University
Ranchi-834008 (Jharkhand)

Preface

Ethical issues in biology and medicine form an important part in ethical discussion these days. Biomedical ethics, as we cryptically call it, becomes more interesting when we consider some value-laden issues in the Indian context. I was engaged in considering some of these issues during the Major Research Project Work funded by the UGC during 1997 to 2000. The above issues were considered for elaborate discussion in the year 1998 while I covered the moral opinions of some doctors, nurses, the patients, and families of bereaved people, lawyers, philosophers and many others. The readers of volumes One and Two of the Series of *Practical and Professional Ethics* have no doubt why I cared so much for the moral opinions of the people mentioned above. For one thing, I still have no doubt that euthanasia, abortion and many value-laden cases need not be analyzed purely on the basis of what has been written about these issues in a number of books available to us. Truly, many health care professionals and ethicists have realized the truth and have come forward in their work-fields, particularly in hospitals, to face many value-laden issues in medicine and biology with the common people, who appear as patients, their families and the lawyers and the lawmakers and policy-makers as well. Hopefully, in our medical and other educational institutions some people are aware of the value of value-resolutions in the field of biomedicine with a range of people and some have tried to find out moral courses of action in our institutions not being isolated from the common milieu. I would put here my experiences as an ethicist who takes up the task of constructing a Biomedical Ethics which does not merely inquire into the theoretical aspects in this field but gets involved in the real dynamics of value-resolution so that our society gets a glimpse of what *people* (health care professionals inclusive), feel about the moral courses of action desirable to be performed in the face of moral crises like euthanasia, abortion and many other issues.

It has been a painstaking but pleasant experience to talk to people about these issues. After I have finished the work, I feel deep respect for a number of health care professionals and other concerned people. I have seen that even the busiest doctor in my city would immediately call me in their chamber to listen to what exactly I wanted to do as soon as I sent a chit on which I wrote: "Purpose: Academic". I therefore expect to unfold the value of a dynamic biomedical ethics in this work.

Contents

Introduction

We had a cute black puppy called *Kutuwa* (derived from kutta or dog) when we lived in the Kathara coalfield. So far as I remember, I picked it from a bush as its mother left it alone for reasons unknown. It looked so beautiful and gestured and played so cutely that the entire family fell in its love, though frankly we were never great pet lovers. We never had one before *Kutuwa* was adopted. I was in class seven at that time; studies did not mean so crazily careeristic to us. We had plenty of time to fondle the puppy, wash it, play with it or just freak with it in a lazy afternoon when others took a nap. After a few months of bonhomie and great care, *Kutuwa* fell ill. It started vomiting frequently and within two days it started dangling on feet, not able to run or even stand properly. It looked rickety, dull and in mute pain. We had no clue to such sickness, nor did the sympathetic but untrained local chemist, who gave medicines, had any idea. Even the professional doctor in the local hospital having no vet-experience though, was of any help. Yet, we all tried our best, the chemist and the doctor gave medicines. The whole neighbourhood soon came to know that something was wrong. My notorious darling friends rallied around us but *Kutuwa* left us all on the fourth day at about seven in the evening. The whole family (except my father) wept profusely. My friends too were in tears and we took funeral in good numbers to the nearby field, dug a deep hole, put *Kutuwa* in eternal sleep to finish the rituals. Then I stood up, with some dug out soil, put it in a piece of paper and returned home. I vowed in front of all gods and goddesses available to us (thanks to my mother), that "I will be a doctor and treat helpless creatures like *Kutuwa*".

Years passed, I started doing well in biology which encouraged me in my goal in life. This continued up to the intermediate classes (standard XI and XII); till I discovered that I was not as good with biology as I assumed. The intricacies of the subject soon demystified me with all the tenterhooks of Islets Langerhan and Golgi Bodies posing nightmare. So I gave up the vow, *Kutuwa* was a forgotten story. I did my doctorate in Philosophy instead of being a doctor, when proudly my lovers called me Doctor till one of my acquaintances, who was another Doctor of Physics, reminded me that we are "good for nothing doctors" whereas physicians are "good for something doctors".

In the year 1997 or a few years before it, when ethics entangled me badly in its love, Gods and Goddesses thought to give me another chance to keep my vow. I started biology and medicine with "good for something people" seriously again, but this time, I was equipped with ethics to meet the scalpel. What did I intend to do? An answer to this question now amounts to Biomedical Ethics hopefully, not another book in the vast sea of information in this field.

My intentions in this book are to clarify first of all that an ethical discussion in the fields of biology and medicine is justified, that is, biomedical ethics makes sense within the field of ethics. It is also important to clarify that biomedical ethics is better understood within Professional Ethics having close relationship with practical, sub-professional and environmental ethics. In Chapter 2 of the book, I shall deal with some other crucial problems, mostly theoretical as well as the problem of models of value-resolution in biology and medicine. In the next few chapters I shall consider the value-laden practical problems of health care, nursing, caring high risk group of people, issues in reproductive technologies, organ donation and transplantation, euthanasia and abortion for ethical resolution with the concerned parties. The chapters are built up on the basis of theoretical information, moral dialogues, and analysis of dialogues and construction of decision-making rules. Most of the time views of the patients and their relatives shall be shielded for identity on their request. A conclusive chapter shall focus on the issues of law, medicine and ethics, and teaching ethics and biomedical ethics to the prospective doctors and professional doctors.

To complete this work I relied heavily on my dear students Mr. Rajendra Kumar and Mr. Purushottam Kumar who carried me to distant places on bikes to meet people for ethical dialogues and for interviews. I also thank many philosophy students and teachers of my department in Ranchi University to arrange moral dialogues. I got immense help from a number of doctors, nurses, missionaries, lawyers, patients and their relatives who talked to me or who participated in these discourses. I must thank the staff of the National Library, particularly Mr. G Kumarappa for his kind cooperation. I am deeply indebted to Mr. Sushil Kumar Ankan, a philosopher friend, who does excellent work in sound recording in his studio. Most of the poorly recorded cassettes have been retrieved by him for a re-recording painstakingly. I thank Mr. Sanjay Singh for carefully typing the manuscript and the Concept Publishing Company for publishing the work.

1

Nature and Justification of Biomedical Ethics

In both the works on Practical Ethics and Professional Ethics and Environmental Ethics often referred to as Vols. 1 and 2 of the Series of *Practical and Professional Ethics*, I have said that Ethics as a branch of Philosophy is ever growing as it percolates in several areas for countering value-laden problems because such problems are not either purely theoretical or practical or both; they are rather queer ones, needing much care of the people of ethical wisdom. These problems, apart from other things, raise distinct questions of moral—should, ought, desirable, duty, right and obligation. Another important feature of these value-laden problems is that they are not easily resolved by dogmatic opinion or opinions of a person or persons in a society or societies, they rather amount to heated disagreements before some kind of agreement could be crystallized, which is, however, a matter of constant scrutiny in times to come. This is not to say that nothing is objectively valid in time and tide as sometimes, some people prefer dead bodies palatable and at other instances not. The question is, even if objectively speaking we agree that dead bodies do not make a good food for any of us at any time, anywhere for simple scientific grounds of health and hygiene (even at the face of the fact that at times of crises, food is a distant cry, people are after a grain flowing in a dirty nullah), how do we *reach such agreement?* Naturally the disagreement-agreement scenario in ethical matters is not as simple as we think them to be because more often than not people reject moral guardians as outclasses and ask for some respect towards general consensus. If this be true, I have argued that ethical matters in our societies make good cases of dynamicity on the part of those caring for such matters.

Ethics as such is thus dynamic, as I have argued. Practical ethics and professional ethics ask for great dynamicity, therefore, though analyzing moral arguments, finding interplay of norms of ethics, the peculiar character of ethical language when speakers of such language are at effective and affective best, and the grandeur of human virtues and values, are all very important. Nothing is different when we consider some value-laden practical problems in the fields of biology and medicine, most fondly called, biomedical ethical problems or simply, bioethics. In case of my adolescent love for pet-street-dogs and its premature death (mentioned in Preface), an ethicist like me who does not necessarily know the details of biomedical intricacies, would still in the capacity of a concerned person having ethical experiences ask: Was it proper for pet-keepers like myself to not to go through the initial and the following check-ups necessary for keeping a pet in a decent hygienic way? Was it proper for an industrial township providing well enough health care facilities for people but no care to provide at least one veterinary surgeon and vet-medicines? Both questions are related but different. Apparently for a commoner in India, such ethically oriented questions do not make much sense because dogs and horses are never as important as humans are, and the problem of distribution of health care facilities for the beings and things on which people depend are thought to be secondary. Sometimes such problems are taken as problems of affluence rather than ethical. The 'ought' for the caretaker and for the distributor nevertheless are important questions because for a poor and for an affluent person, dogs, monkeys and horses are important beings emotionally, practically and even theoretically. Is it not good for me whose father was not even a middle-class worker in a coalfield to keep a dog? Or, is it not desirable that poorest of the poor keeps a monkey with him or a dog or a snake, share his shabby bits of food with pets, depend on them to eke out a living and still the person thinks that nothing is great about the society who does not make much distinction between a dog and a man when it comes to distribution of means of welfare? This way we may go on peeling the scales of problems surrounding myself and my pet on the one hand and the welfare and distribution of pleasures on the other hand. The problems are not merely practical; they are "value-laden" as well. But why call such problems "biomedical" or more correctly, "biomedical-ethical" or "bioethical"?

Any ethical concern about matters pertaining to "life" on earth in several forms should be called "life ethics" or "bioethics".

However, special reference to ethical concern in "medical" matters or what may be called "medical ethics" is a little different from "bioethics", as in the former case, we are particularly dealing with ethical aspects involved in the medical science in which doctor-patient relationship as well as the care-taking units' and patients' relationship are important. It is not necessary to include within this area the different concerns about non-human animals' and care-taking units' relationship because for that we have another science called the veterinary science wherein several ethical matters are important. One realizes at this point that all forms of non-human life has not been well covered under "medical ethics" because non-human animals do not fill up the entire body of life-forms on earth and for that reason ethical questions relating to non-human life should be considered separately. Hence, "medical ethics", "veterinary ethics" and "animal ethics" are different ways to know about ethical concerns about "life" (bio) in general. Obviously many interesting and important ethical questions with regard to humans, non-human animals and non-animal life forms (if that is a sensible term) constitutes what we broadly know as "bioethics" or ethical inquiries pertaining to "life". "Bioethics" is thus "life ethics" in the real sense of the term, which is in fact, in the *common parlance, referred to as biomedical ethics*. Nevertheless, "medical" as conjoined to "life", qualifies "life" to a great degree and restricts our discussion. For simplicity, one might speak of "bioethics" but the term cannot be taken as equivalent to "biomedical ethics" or "medical ethics", which I prefer to use here. Truly speaking, a reference to "bioethics" would happily include veterinary ethics, ethics relating to the vegetable kingdom, microscopic and ultramicroscopic life forms as well as medical and nursing ethics but I take the liberty to discuss biomedical ethics that leaves out many issues related to numerous 'life-forms'. Biomedical ethics include ethics of care and ethics relating to entire care-taking unit of humans, non-human animals and non-animal life. Naturally, it includes ethics of allocation and distribution of means of care for these beings on earth and in many cases means of effective management and/or eradication of certain beings (viruses, microbes and others) because they are arguably *evil* ones. Biomedical ethics also includes ethics of experimentation and research with several life forms for effective care and management of flourishing human life on earth. This will naturally include operations, organ transplantations, cloning, termination of life (of so-called valuable life forms and not viruses), dissection of non-human living beings for educational purposes, manipulations with genes, banking of potential life forms and life savers and also our dealing with humans in vegetative as well as insane conditions. It will no doubt include the intricate politics, economics and business (all involving ethical scrutiny), with human life and for human life. Biomedical ethics is, therefore, Pandora's Box; if we shut it, there is no wonder for us to be revealed, and if we open it, we will be soon awestruck by the complexities involving us.

Biomedical ethics, which is not so broad a field, is still extremely interesting if we delve deeper into it. Though it is predominantly anthropocentric or human-centred ethical discussion, in reality, it is something more. In one sense, it is about relation of the sick and the healthy as well as many perceptions and challenges within this risk-relationship. It is also relation among the living, the dying and the dead. It covers a queer realm of death and life and our duties, obligations and responsibilities with regard to the living, the dying and the dead. At times, it is also a relation of the living and the call for the right to die as well as for the right to life. It covers the legal mesh which is never beyond ethical inquiries. There is no doubt therefore that biomedical ethics or simply medical ethics is as intricate a matter as the ethical concern in "life" in general. Yet, several transverse discussions enable us to discover that "bio" conjoined to "medical" amounts to consideration of matters of human life as related to other life forms and it will be overlooking this truth if we believe that "biomedical" amounts to matter relating to doctor, patient, treatment, caretaking people and allocation and distribution of resources for care. Naturally, "biomedical" ethics takes care of such ethical matters which arise from an interface of the sick, the healthy, the doctor and other caretakers and the non-human animals as well as other life forms. For instance, in case of our ethical concern for experimentation on monkeys for non-cosmetic medical tests for treating the humans, apart from the patient and health caretakers and distributors, we include our non-human ethical concerns in experimentations. Even for medical education, in voluntary deployment of donors or subjects for tests, experiments and demonstrations, particularly the animals raise ethical questions though here we are broadly concerned with something *beyond* the sick-healthy relationship. More interesting cases may be taken from use of vegetable life forms for treatment of the sick humans with an added dimension of policies and economies involved in such matters as is the case when in our times margosa and turmeric are aggressively fought for patenting of herbal drugs though the bone of contention is saving life by curing maladies. And the question of adequate medical use of these herbs in connection to some patent bluffs does raise serious ethical concerns in medical treatment. The belligerence among alternative treatments and medicines, the bashing of homoeopathy or ayurved as trash by the allopath are no less medical ethical matters for consideration. Hence, it will be too narrow to say that biomedical ethics amounts to the ethics of treatment and management of the sick humans by healthy care takers and nothing else. Broadly speaking, therefore, "biomedical ethics" with which we are concerned here is not synonymous to bioethics, but it does involve ethical questions pertaining to the treatment and management of sick persons by health care professionals, their interaction with the families of sick people, the society at large and also consideration of ethic of the involvement of non-human life forms in such treatment and management. Keeping these things in mind, I shall stick to the use of "biomedical ethics" rather than "bioethics". The moral questions taken hereafter for resolution are thus involving health care professionals, sick people, their families, the common people of our societies, the decision-makers and distributors as well as animals and vegetarians mostly competent as means for our medical welfare.

In fact, Van Rensselaer Potter first used the term "bioethics" in his seminal work *Bioethics: Bridge to the Future* (1971) in the introductory part (pp. vii-viii) to refer to ethical issues pertaining to human population and environment at large. My analysis of "bio" in "bioethics" reflects this truth but Potter has finally restricted the use of the notion to refer to ethical issues in health care, which truly speaking amounts to "biomedical ethics", as I have said. Nevertheless, the narrow use of "medical ethics" or "biomedical ethics" is old enough in which the term "medical" as we have seen, refers to anyone involved in health care. We have to remember that even this use of the term is broad enough as in medical ethics gradually we have restricted our discussion to the physician or the doctor treating sick people. Due to this, Robert Veatch in his work *A Theory of Medical Ethics* (1981) has demarcated the *broad* and the *narrow* uses of "medical" in "medical ethics". If one keeps in mind the other sense in which "bio" may be affixed in the "medical" in the broadest connotation perhaps, we may say that "biomedical ethics" may be used as broader, broad and narrow senses but not broadest as "bioethics" is used. In this sense, more loosely spoken or narrow sense of "medical ethics" is nothing but "physician ethics". However, "health care ethics" is broader; involving not merely physicians but nurses as well. Interestingly, we may go on speaking separately about "nursing ethics" having different connotation from "health care ethics" and even "physician ethics". However, "physician ethics" comes within "professional ethics" as well as "health care ethics", nursing being a "sub-profession" (see Vol. 1) is within "sub-professional ethics" but not outside "health care ethics". "Health care ethics" is therefore an amalgam of issues considered from ethical perspective which involves professionals, sub-professionals and non-professionals. Shortly we shall find that "practical ethics" is inseparably linked to this complex whole called "health care ethics". In fact, medical ethics and biomedical ethics in their respective broad and broader sense are inseparably related to professional, sub-professional and practical ethics. As I have used "bio" in "biomedical ethics" broadly, there should not be much hassle in its acceptance as ethical concerns about matters relating to physicians and many other parties that form a complex group with regard to health care.

Biomedicine as we now understand it, in association to ethics is essentially *interdisciplinary* needing information from both fields of biology and medicine. Many people are of the opinion that ethical and philosophical interests in biology and medicine have enriched human wisdom. There are people who say that it is biomedicine which has relieved ethics and philosophy of its hackneyed theoretic hangover. Anyway the point is not one of greatness of biomedical ethics because in any case, we have to go for an evaluation of the same for its value in civil societies.

Biomedical ethics is an old field as I understand it because history of ancient Greek and Indian philosophy is punctuated with such interdisciplinary studies. Almost all of us and the prospective doctors know that there was someone called Hypocrite, Charaka and Sushruta and many others who took some interest in the ethical inquiry of medical matters. Yet, the rise and growth of Biomedical Ethics in our times is marked by phenomenal writings in this field during the late 60s up to mid-70s, particularly in the UK, USA and Canada. In the western world, the dominion of the Christian biomedical thinkers as well as other thinkers added some unique flavour to these writings. One can easily find widespread theological ethical orientation in these works in the 70s in particular. With this spurt, the biomedical discussion has grown worldwide; India does not lag behind. We have reports of biomedical ethical discussions in some institutions like the All India Institute of Medical Sciences (AIIMS) and Central Institute of Psychiatry (CIP). In the United States the growth of biomedical science has been phenomenal, championed by the Hasting Centre (also its Report is worth considering), Kennedy Institute, Society for Health and Human Values, American Philosophical Association and many more. In the UK, the *British Medical Journal (BMJ)* and the *Journal of Medicine and Philosophy* in the USA have contributed substantially to the growth of biomedical ethics. Today we have a number of institutes, centers, societies and journals contributing to its growth. The number of books published in this field is of anyone's envy. Teaching biomedical ethics is not a great passion in India, as is not writing in this field, though in the USA and the UK, it has become almost a national passion, which I respect. However, I trash the idea that it is face-saving for philosophy and philosophers who are believed to be on life-saving system. Mary B. Mahowald reports in her essay that: "Recently, a new kind of expert in biomedical ethics has emerged. This is the individual who is fully prepared in philosophy and in his or her health care speciality... For example, Howard Brody, a physician-philosopher"[1]. Later on I would like to comment on some such "experts" whom I do not take as positively contributing to biomedical ethics, if we have decided about the nature and method of such interdisciplinary study because these people tend to act as ethics-engineers in an artificial manner. Last but not the least is to mention about the publication of Encyclopaedia of Bioethics (1978) which is full of value-laden biomedical issues and suggestions for their resolution.

Without going into the issues taken under biomedical ethics, we have to further clarify the sense in which ethical concern about biomedicine is different from biomedical basis of ethics. There must be significant features of both clarifying their nuances. This is needed for clarification of the sense of biomedical ethics itself or else, under popular opinion we will believe that ethical concerns in biology and medicine are owing to the truism that ethics is based on biology. But this is gross misunderstanding. First, let us consider what amounts to the biological basis of ethics and whether or not ethics is really based on biology. It is natural to think that in the vast teeming nature, what I sometimes call "ecological community" (see vols. 1 and 2), man has come to existence or has evolved, grown, flourished and fizzled out. Without the basic biological conditions prevailing in nature, man could not have evolved and nor flourished. In the course of human evolution and its manifold growth, it showed signs of ethical thinking, decision-making as well as unethical thinking and decision-making. All these things cannot have come as a bolt from the blue as our acumen to decide about the desirable and the good or the undesirable and the evil owe much to our conditions in nature. Hence, throughout the world, human acumen to think, decide and act ethically (and unethically) is deeply related to the biological conditions in and around the beings. The problem is why other animals were not able to have such acumen when they had favourable conditions to evolve? The question is much like why did we have human language and animals failed to have that, though language may be taken at present universally among animals of higher degree of physical and mental evolution. We are not sure whether the honesty of dog is instinctive or, is ethically intended, still we can safely say that the natural environmental conditions apart, the non-human animals live an entirely different form of life than the humans, which is crucial to our having unique ethical acumen in the mother nature, while others do not have it. Hence, just for the truth that all animals are part and parcel of nature, the biological factors notwithstanding, ethicality is simply not a matter of being one among the existential in nature, it is something more. Our sense of good, desirable, rights, justice and so on are unique to our *form of life* which is distinctively marked by *complex interaction* we have with humans, non-human beings and also many things in nature, and the resulting *moral reasons* that emanate by virtue of our evolved mental abilities. Hopefully, non-human animals, though having almost equally complex form of life (in case of domestic animals, they are deeply related to human ways of living), still the moral reasons, analytic powers and language use make them essentially different from us. Hence, human ethicality does have a strong biological basis but that is not all, the way humans live and the way they think, reason, analyze and use language, make them the unique ethical beings they are. This is to say that though ethics as a *subject* in philosophy has biological origin; it is independently based, the ethical ways of thinking about the right and the good and the actions performed thereby does have a biological basis. This needs some clarification as "ethics" within philosophy (and philosophy itself) is not merely dealing with what is right and good, it reasons with *why* something is right and good, *what* is the *meaning* of "right" and "good", why something that is the basis of right and good is itself worth considering and *how* something that is right and good should be achieved in the society in the face of widespread disagreements. Clearly, the subject called "ethics" is not merely dealing with the ways in which we come to *know* about right and good, which is nevertheless a matter of our being in biological conditions, it deals with many other things where our individual and collective thinking, rationalizing, universalizing, criticism, analysis, reasoning, refutation, disagreements, agreements, deciding and acting become extremely vital, and these contribute to our unique *non-biological conditions* or better said, *conditions transcending the biotic life and the natural environmental conditions*. This is one crucial point in realizing that ethics within philosophy cannot be said to be wholly based on biology though our ethical knowledge stems from certain experiences in biotic nature, and for that matter only in a special sense, ethics is based on biology. Here, "ethics" is not "ethics as a branch of philosophy" rather *human ethical experience and knowledge* of the right and the good etc. which is based on the biotic system in which humans thrive. We can now realize that biology is a subject essentially different from ethics as a subject and it will be extremely fertile thinking that as biology deals with natural entities in a special way, it does so because humans are so ethical or good in such thinking. Or, to imagine that ethical language and normative thinking is owing to the fact that we are natural entities and the special science of such entities tell us why we use such language, why such language is true and meaningful and why teleology and deontology should be accepted as they are or why they should be rejected for such and such reasons. There is no doubt that the old belligerence between egoism and altruism as ethical thesis acting more often than not as first principles of morality or the basis of value judgments, have their own biological truths, that is, they must have come from human beings' selection of value of self or others in the society for existence, flourishing and welfare. Truly, these overreaching generalizations of wise people must have strong empirical claims to withstand belligerence but equally true is that the method of generalization needs to be logically or at least heuristically justified, when biology is thus replaced by definite logical reasons. Moreover, choosing one principle and not choosing another one, the smothering of moral tensions leading to decisions and actions are neither emotive nor biological; they are backed up by our moral reasons or moral arguments. These matters are thus testimony to transcendence of biological principles or biological facts or phenomena. One may argue that the so-called "reasons" are not in the domain of a ghost in the machine because to know about their possibility is to know about basic biological evolution of mind, its disposition, and its several functions and so on. Alas, the first lesson we got in our preliminary classes in philosophy and in psychological basis of ethics is that in these fields we do not worry about the evolution, constitution and function of mind and powers of rationality, we are more concerned about the nature, role, extent and usefulness of reason in moral matters. We are here not to know about what happens when we provide moral reasons or how does it happen in us, rather, what effect does reason have in moral matters and the strengths and weaknesses of the logic inherent in such reasons. Hence, biology might have capacities to unfold the empirical aspects of many moral theses but ethics *per se* is much beyond it. It is due to this that the sciences of biology and medicine or biomedicine or biotechnology are essentially different from the ethical scrutiny of biology, medicine, biomedicine, biotechnology and so on. To confuse biomedical ethics with biological basis of ethics is unfounded. It is a confusion of failing to understand ethical discussions pertaining to biology and medical and biological talk relevant in an understanding of why ethical experience and knowledge of the good and the right is but natural for all humans in the world. As ethics-talk being relevant to biology does not prove that ethics is the foundation or basis of biology, biological-talk as relevant to moral knowledge does not prove that biology is the basis of ethics. Any obstinate logic would rather prove that we do not know what biology and ethics are.

To justify what has been said just now (and to show finally that biology cannot be the basis of ethics), we have to consider "obstinate" views for a thorough analysis. This has been done wonderfully by Peter Singer in *The Expanding Circle* (1981). He shows us how Edward Wilson in his much touted work on *Sociobiology* had justified that socio-biological explanation of ethical matters is the only sound way. For him matters like ethical good and evil depends on our analysis of human emotion control centre in the brain. Reading the book painstakingly Singer comments that: "Although Wilson is clear that *sociobiology* should make a dramatic difference to ethics, he is regrettably less clear about exactly what difference it makes. For the next 500 pages of *Sociobiology* there is nothing to suggest how biology can explain ethics "at all depths" until in the final chapter of the book, Wilson abruptly suggests that perhaps "the time has come for ethics to be removed temporarily from the hands of the philosophers and biologicized"[2]. Whatever Singer thinks about Wilson, we have to find out what is so irrelevant in Wilson's views. Wilson thinks that the institutions which have helped in generalization of deontological principle of morality should be better traced to the emotive centre of their own hypothalamic-limbic systems. Wilson is exactly worried about what a biologist should worry about but he completely forgets that *qua* ethicists we are not at all interested in deciphering "what goes in our brain when we generalize duty as the first principle" rather, we are interested in knowing what Wilson thinks about the nature and role of motives, intentions, emotions in ethical decision-making and actions and what are the bearings of speakers' and hearers' emotions in the explication of meaning of ethical language. Wilson must know that what happens in us while we intend to do our duties is different from analysis of meaning of "duty" and the connection of intending and moral acting or doing or doing for the intrinsic value of doing something. His thinking that on the bases of evolutionary testimonies we can show why young people are likely to be egoists than older people who are altruists may have some truth which must be evidently probable as all scientific truths are but such discoveries do not to the least prove that, therefore, biology is the bases of ethics. What at best it shows is that there are some empirical bases of why we speak of egoism and altruism as ethical thesis. Equally true is that there are empirical bases to say why we are neither egoists nor altruists but something else. Well, Wilson seems to uphold "ethical pluralism" in his book for he must have biological basics going right in his thought process but when he says that such pluralism shows evolutionary approach in ethics as self-evident, is palpable confusion because rather than evolutionism, it is complex *ethical ways of living and interacting* that turns out to be truly the empirical basis of "ethical pluralism" as a valid thesis. Wilson perhaps did not have another idea that ethical disagreement situations in ethical resolution and the likely agreement giving way to resolution justifies pluralism rather than the monolithic structure of normative ethics and its application (see vols. 1 & 2). In fact, Wilson has been thoroughly mesmerized by biological findings evident in evolutionism and neurological explanations so much so that he forgot the basic *category difference* between these *scientific thesis and ethics*. He must have several confusions about ethicality, morality and ethics as well.

Wilson is at pains in *On Human Nature* to show further that ethic of sex is based on biological understanding, that is, what is inherent in our genes. This is laughing I must say because the ethic of sex, like that of ethic of homosexuality boils down to theoretic and practical churnings within the realms of normative and practical ethics, as well as within the discussions of moral virtues and values and not to our genes. The reality is that "what is in our genes" may be or may not be useful in unravelling why some of us are homosexuals or gays but it cannot be useful in showing why some people argue that such acts are ethically desirable and undesirable and the way we come to resolve the ethical impasse in gay rights etc. Wilson has to realize that it is perfectly sensible in ethics to argue for and against sexual rights of sections of people but it is insensible in ethics to search "what is in genes" that "we are homosexuals or think it is good". Suppose some day genetic research reveals that for such and such chemistry in genes we *justify* that homosexuality is ethically good and some call it bad, still in ethics we would transcend the glorious discovery to enquire "on what ethical basis is homosexuality good or bad or it is not a matter of ethical good and bad" and we shall continue to try to resolve the moral crises. So the genetic machinery in us cannot be the basis of our ethical venture about biological matter and for that reason ethic of biology is distinct from biological basis of ethics. Wilson should now realize that any amount of depth study of biology and its bearings on ethical experiences we have cannot justify a valid moral principle or code which is universal. When Wilson speaks of (a) the cardinal value of diverse gene pools, (b) the cardinal value of gene pools, and (c) the cardinal value of mammalian nature of the Homo sapiens for the universal rights movement, he forgets that the said cardinal values are for the safeguard of a thinking, rather a morally thinking species but not for the sake of empowering the said species to think morally in the way or in many ways. Biology cannot empower humans to think and act morally or to become ethicists. Biology cannot help sustain ethics as a subject either.

Wilson and many others are enthusiastic about Darwinian evolutionary thesis being the basis of ethical principle we call "evolutionism". This is to say that whatever evolves is itself good and for that reason ethical evolution of human beings and societies should be judged as good. However, Wilson is not emphatic about this point. Still, I must stress that the evolution of the Homo sapiens as those caring for moral values does not prove either that biology is the basis of ethics or that evolutionary thesis is the first principle in morality. The fact that we have evolved as those talking about ethical matters apart from other things is to forget that we are palpable nuisance makers, trouble shooting, grossly unethical beings, which hopefully we shall remain in our cloned versions possibly in the future. Yet, we shall remain talkative about why gross unethicality is undesirable. But that shows that evolutionary thesis itself is not universally valid as we argue strongly against such thesis as of any value in ethics. The illogic of the thesis is what the crux of ethics is because ethics is greatly concerned with weighing the logic of such thesis, which is not based on biology. However, Singer thinks that if there are some biological theses which are relevant to ethical decision-making, they should be given some importance within ethics but that still does not justify that biology is the basis of ethics because more important in ethics is to show the ways in which we can or cannot contest the so-called biological thesis as relevant to ethics. Equally true is that within ethics we still argue forcefully about the relevance of ethical scrutiny of biological matters. To weigh these arguments is perhaps distinctive to ethics, which biology in no way helps in doing. We shall soon take up the problem of the justification of ethical-talk in biomedicine; shortly before that we should ask with regard to Wilson's position that someway do we really have justification of ethics *per se* on biological basis?

Wilson thinks that biology can sufficiently disprove the existing ethical thesis thus establishing new ones. Hence, biology can make phenomenal changes in our ethical opinions about certain value-laden issues like gay rights and homosexuality. It is due to this that rejecting homosexuality as having any ethic on the ground that it is unnatural to human nature and thus undesirable has been completely replaced by the biological thesis that homosexuality is in fact very natural to human nature. Does this prove that biology has changed the ethical scrutiny of homosexuality? Certainly not, because even if it be true that homosexuality is natural and not unnatural biologically speaking, it has not changed the raging questions of desirable and undesirable. In fact the moral disagreement regarding this matter is not merely due to thinking the act as natural or unnatural to man, it is owing to differences in opinion about the independent ethical reasons to judge the action right or wrong or good or bad.

Peter Singer draws another charge against Wilson's misconception which has been put in another way by me in Vols. 1 and 2 of the Series. We ask Wilson whether or not he understands the role of biological science in shaping some universal principles of morality, which are often believed to be systematic accounts of our moral intuitions? In fact the said moral intuitions which we have for instance about utilitarianism are systematized in that shape not by virtue of one or more scientific findings like those in biology. The point that we are "naturally" inclined to maximize pleasures for more and more people may be biologically true but that testimony does not go for or against utilitarianism. Similarly, our "nature" being testimony to be inclined to homosexuality is not the basis of a systematized universal moral intuition of egoistic hedonism. What I have said in particular in this matter is that the moral experience and knowledge we acquire in this world owe much to the interactions with the biotic life or what is ecological community but such moral experiences and knowledge need systematization by virtue of rigorous justifications, which is studied under metaethics and not biology. Hence, moral theories as overreaching first principles do not owe to biological science but they do owe to the experience we have in the ecological community. There is a difference, Mr. Wilson, between depending on biotic life forms and depending on biology. Ethics is categorically different from biology; therefore, it does not logically depend on it for justification of crucial thesis. Peter Singer supports it in these words: "science is outside ethics, the scientific study of the origin of our ethical judgment is a fulcrum on which we can rest our critical lever. In itself, science cannot compel us to abandon a principle – a fulcrum is not a force – but coupled with a commitment to *rationality* (my italics), it can provide leverage against basic ethical principles"[3]. And he wonders: "If all our ethical principles can be shown to be relics of our evolutionary or cultural history, are they all equally discredited?"[4]

What both Singer and I have in mind may be put in yet another way (thankfully Singer speaks about it as well); we may ask Mr. Wilson whether or not he is aware of the danger of desiring what ought or should be done, that is, what is morally desirable from what are the facts or instances or concrete testimonies in nature? My position is that any moral theory as found in systematized forms by virtue of rigorous thinking of some wise men do not drop from the blue, they have empirical bases. Even a champion phenomenological ethical thinker would first need to exist along with the intricate patterns of existence on the whole or else nothing emanates from even "pure intentionality". But this does not amount to say that only if there were factual evidences in nature, we *derive* (logically) ethical ought or should. The reason is that even if a common, uneducated person has experiences of what goes around him or her and imagines or intuits that this is the way things *should* be done now, the said intuition of the "should" does not amount to any theory, which is applied by that illiterate person in his or her life to do what he thinks he should do. This is because he finds that what he imagines as the standard of doing in life is judged as vulgar or immoral by others, and soon the personal moral likes or inclinations of "should" fizzles out. Or else, the person sometimes overcomes social pressures in his lifetime to overpower the several wrong moral notions prevalent in society to prove that even a group intuition of moral "should" is immoral. Social life, of which moral life is a part, does not crystallize "should" or "ought" from mere facts, opinions and predilections, the "ought" is often universally derived either by virtue of rigorous *moral reasoning* and *moral arguments* after *resolution of stiff moral disagreements* among people. In any case, even if universal moral theories are reflected in opinion of uncommon people who depend much on facts for such opinions, they are shaped as standards about moral "ought" and "should" by transcending facts to enter into the realms of reasons, arguments and consensus. I strongly believe that there is no "pure intuition" as is there no "pure intention" helping us to derive *ought from is* because finding moral "ought" is not a matter of inductive or deductive reasoning, neither is it a matter of thinking *a priori* or stark empirical experiences; much really depends on transcending strict rules of logic, embracing different *informal arguments*, *heuristics*, and most importantly, going through *systematic scrutiny of moral dialogues*. Hence, I support Singer when he says: "No science is ever going to discover ethical premises inherent in our biological nature, because ethical premises are not the kind of thing discovered by scientific investigation. We do not find our ethical premises in our biological nature"[5].

I am grateful to Singer in pressing an absurdity in Wilson's view by showing the blatant *logical inconsistency* involved in accepting biology as the basis of ethics. Analyzing what Wilson has argued in terms of proving moral "ought" as logically derived from factual "is", Singer shows that the *premise* of the argument, "our genes came from a common pool and will return to a common pool", which is *factual* (biologically based), is the basis to derive the *conclusion* which is moral, "therefore we ought not to do anything which imperils the common gene pool". However, we know that without introducing a moral premise in the given argument, from a factual premise, no ethical conclusion (about ought) can be logically derived. Hence, Wilson's argument is fallacious. Singer imagines that had Wilson introduced a *second premise* in the argument having a moral (ought) element therein, still the said conclusion will not hold good, that is, if the "second premise" is: "We ought not to do anything which imperils the long-term survival of our genes", is not factual; rather the introduction of "ought" here has given it a different status, which is open to further logical scrutiny and also disagreement. The problem is why *should* we *not* imperil the common gene pool? Wilson gives us no biological or moral argument here. Let me add here that had Wilson given a biological or factual proof, it would further not justify the "ought" element in the premise (following our first argument) and had he given a moral proof, it is a matter of controversy for it begs a moral standard as the starter, which is itself dubitable and not self-proved. On the basis of all these arguments I would like to say what Singer asserts nicely: "Neither evolutionary theory, nor biology, nor science as a whole can provide the ultimate premises of ethics. Biological explanations of ethics can only perform the negative role of making us think again about moral intuitions which we take to be self evident moral truths but can be explained in evolutionary terms"[6]. Hence, we believe that "Unless there is a rational component to ethics that we can use to defend at least one of our fundamental ethical principles, the free use of biological and cultural explanations would leave us in a state of deep moral subjectivism"[7]. Thus we would end as Singer did: "reason is not powerless. On the *collective level* (my italics), once we hence begun to justify our conduct publicly, reason leads us to develop and expand our moral concerns, drawing us on towards an objective point of view… The shape of human ethical systems is an outcome of the attempt of human societies to cope with this tension between *collective reasoning* (my italics)"[8].

With this we come to an end of confusion, that is, confusion about the nature of biomedical ethics. If such confusions are nurtured, we are unclear about what exactly we are attempting to know and explain. We come to know that biomedical ethics deals with some such issues arising out of human enterprises in biology and medicine which raise distinct questions of ethical desirability, good, right and just. We shall not deal with the range of these issues now because we have still not faced the challenge of "justification" of biomedical ethics. Many among us might argue (as many philosophers would) that even if we have successfully shown that ethics does not depend on biology and biomedical ethics does not amount to an ethical adventure (or misadventure!) which is based only on biological findings and theories for its success, the entire effort understood to be within the field of ethics is completely mistaken. There is either no point in an ethical scrutiny of biomedical issues, which are often called "value-laden issues" by the ethicists or other parties or, there is no point in a biomedical scientific scrutiny of the relevance of value-questions or ethical questions arising within biology and medicine. The point is that biomedical ethics cannot be justified as sensible either within ethics or within biological and medical sciences. This is a serious challenge. If we do not meet it head on successfully we have not "justified" biomedical ethics in any sense. Let us start with the discussion.

In the recent times, people like Gary Stahl and David F. Seedhouse have led to some reactions and over-reactions from biologists, physicians and philosophers because biomedical ethics has been either found as redundant (Stahl) or misconceived (Seedhouse). Both attacks on biomedical ethics, particularly the first one have something to do with what we have already found in the context of Wilson. We would first take up Seedhouse's challenge for it is direct – it is *Against medical ethics: a philosopher's view*[9]. Not only this, in a reply to this paper by Jackie Cassell in the *Journal of the Institute of Medical Ethics* (vol. 24, 1998). Seedhouse himself clarifies in a separate paper that his conception of the misconception prevailing about biomedical ethics should be properly evaluated in the context of his broader perspectives on the matter which has been published during 1986 to 1997[10]. However, we have his broader opinion "against ethics" put together simply and precisely in the above mentioned volume of the Journal (BMJ, pp. 13-17). Let us find what Seedhouse has to say against biomedical ethics. He "characterizes" ethics in these terms: "How best to conduct one's life in the presence of the other lives is the founding question of ethics. Thus, all interventions doctors choose to make in the lives of human beings have ethical content, however apparently trivial or technical the encounter"[11]. Seedhouse seems to have no doubt that his apt characterization of ethics as a field within philosophy is good enough. His interpreters like Cassell do not doubt either because for them "ethics" is concerned with whole of human life as intricately involved with other lives and any actions against another life comes within the ethical scanner, and that all of our actions affecting others though apparently mechanical, does come for an ethical scrutiny. Though I have something to say about this *characterization of ethics* itself, let us listen more to Seedhouse. Before this characterization of ethics Seedhouse has made *two claims*: The *first* is that it is impossible to distinguish the ethical from the non-ethical when we are concerned about medical care of living beings, and for that matter, medical ethics makes no sense as an independent branch of study. Hence, one misconception has been sorted out regarding medical ethics, which in Stahl's parlance must be happily taken as "redundant". The *second* claim is that long ethical tradition as developed by ethical or moral philosophers is one of establishment of theories or norms, which medical ethics fails to do rather goes on blindly taking one such theory or more as true and effective on medical situations as parasitic to moral philosophy. It is not strange that the "characterization" of "ethics" by Seedhouse should be exactly as what he says here because the first claim makes it clear that for him ethics covers concerns of whole of human life, the biomedical concerns inclusive, hence, there is no point in a separate non-ethical study like biomedical ethics. The second claim is not distinct either because for Seedhouse ethics properly so-called is a long story of normativism, which independently covers questions of human life for resolution – why should we need biomedical ethics in addition to it when that is non-moral or better said factual? Now here we are reminded of what Wilson said about biology as basis of ethics, the question is who is putting the horse before the cart? Certainly Wilson was grossly mistaken as Cassell thinks that Seedhouse too is confused by virtue of unwanted commitment to "naturalism". I think we should take on Cassell's criticism, but before that we should give Seedhouse enough opportunity to clarify his position, which he does in reply to Cassell in the above mentioned journal.

For Seedhouse there are two forms of the *ethical*, A and B: where ethical A means "ethical in the sense of having ethical content" and ethical B means "ethical in the sense of having consistent view about what one ought to do in the social world"[12]. Ethical A is nothing but some situations in our life judged for good or bad, right or wrong etc., for they have positive or negative effects on people, beings and things around us. For instance, deliberately disturbing the classroom by a huge sigh or a long sneeze though sighing and sneezing themselves are not matters of moral scrutiny or that they are non-moral. Ethical B on the other hand is to know what is ethical A, intend and decide to act in one way which is ethical and unethical and does so for he or she has enough moral basis for doing so, as and when one decides not to sneeze so long or in a rustic fashion in classroom for it is harmful as well as disturbing to others. If we know ethical A and B, Seedhouse believes that ethical arena stands out to be one of mesh (not mess) of agreement and disagreement for the ways in which ethical life ought to be lived in practice, is open to debate and rarely a consensus could be found, for consensus needs some effort.

If we now reflect on medical ethics in which consideration of good of human health is vital for moral reasons and not for scientific ones merely, "work for health" is "a certain sort of moral endeavour" says Seedhouse. Most important to mention here is that such endeavours do not help us in distinguishing the ethical from the non-ethical because "work for health" is ethical in the sense of ethical A and the sense of being ethical A enable workers in that field to exert seriously for ethical B. And what is important to notice here is that for Seedhouse (or proponents of such view), ethical B calls for normativism or else it is of least possibility. Theories of ethics are thus prerequisites for ethical B. Now, ethical B in medical parlance clearly depends on ethical norms, that is, any ethical concern in medicine or "health work" depends on ethics proper and *not beyond* it. Hence, biomedical ethics makes no sense taken apart from "ethics properly so-called". Unambiguously Seedhouse says: "My idea, in a nutshell, is that health workers should take as much command as they can of the ethical A by committing to an ethical B based on the foundations theory of work for health"[13].

Whatever blatant confusions Seedhouse views like that have shall be mentioned in no less unambiguous terms here but I must mention that the way his views were analyzed by Dr. Cassell and others championing the cause of medical ethics is not pertinent enough. First, Dr. Cassell (as I believe) argues wrongly that Seedhouse's conception of ethical A and B is out of track in so far as there is no pronouncement of which norm (in ethical A) should govern ethical B in case of a doctor in "work". Seedhouse's normative "neutrality" is extremely confusing and defeating as he shows great apathy to the relevance of Kantianism or utilitarianism, for instance. Cassell finds further that Seedhouse's rejection of the ethical and the non-ethical distinction (much unlike Wilson) is unwanted because what is touted "non-ethical" by biomedical ethicists is very much in the realm of the 'ethical A'. However, the non-distinction of the above matters rules out Kant's thesis wherein a stress exclusively on "duty" as clarification of meaning of 'ethical A' as influencing 'ethical B' clearly rules out Seedhouse's "rejection" because

Kant is emphatic about distinguishing all sorts of "works" as those of doctors or others, that is, 'ethical B' out of the realm of the moral if "duty" has not been taken in the sense of the "moral", rather, references are made to 'happiness maximization' and so on. Cassell is of the opinion that Seedhouse's apathy to distinguish the moral and the non-moral is closer to what is said in utilitarianism because this ethical thesis does not hesitate in explaining moral in terms on the basis of non-moral or natural terms and is thus "naturalistic". If Seedhouse is not clear about making this distinction, he would mean what all "naturalists" mean by explaining "medically ethical" or what is non-moral in terms of "ethical properly understood" or simply, moral and thus face all unhappy questions naturalists face. Seedhouse in this sense has great ontological and epistemological problems to face as well, because *per se*, medicine makes the natural and the non-natural distinction clearly, though for that, it does not have to lose its ethical interests. Moreover, if the distinction is not made, the epistemic status of the natural science as distinct from the non-natural discipline, that is, ethics gets blurred.

Still readers are left in the suspicion of what I mean to say because here is for our perusal Gary Stahl's funded research paper *Bioethics: A Redundant Concept* (1998)[14]. Stahl's lengthy paper brings out several points of the "redundancy" of Bioethics and has explained them very well. I will bring out only important ones for a critical study. Stahl argues that "the first sense of redundancy is *ontological*"[15] and "the second sense of redundancy is *judgemental*"[16]. Simple reasons are that it is impossible to do ethics without biology (*cf.* Wilson) and that biomedical issues and ethical issues are not distinguishable, they are the same (*cf.* Seedhouse). The point is that biomedical ethics is a redundant idea because either biology is the basis of ethics and thus sufficient for ethical examinations or ethical issues and biomedical issues are not different. Stahl says that his point is not to reassure this redundancy rather to show the *implications* of such idea of redundancy and thereby come to conclude whether or not the idea itself is justifiable. Stahl makes it clear at the outset that a cluster of so-called bioethical problems like abortion, *In Vitro* tests, experiments on children and animals etc. amounts to "development of the organism in time" or that "whether or not at any given time or stage there is a *person* present". Stahl thinks that if we do not seriously consider the possibility of the ontological priority (or rather fundamentality) of biology over ethics, we are unable to explain the basic question stated above, that is, "who is a person?". Maybe we are unable to explain another basic question, "what is life and death?". Hence, an ethical scrutiny of abortion etc. which we passionately call "biomedical ethical issues" is really "biological" or "biomedical" in essence. I hope our readers must be truly so enriched by the Wilson-Singer debate and Cassell-Seedhouse debate that they easily realize what Stahl wants to press on them. Stahl thinks the dichotomy in redundancy argument could roll together as judgmental redundancy which hints towards nothing but *biomedicine as sufficient* to take care of the ethical questions, the latter is by the first argument shown to be conclusively ontologically based on biology and medicine. Stahl bases his argument about the "judgmental redundancy" on the point that any "judgment" of some biomedical decision as "ethical" or "unethical" depends largely on the factual biological point of clarity of meaning of "health" because biomedicine deals heavily on "health" about which it is concerned primarily. Hence, the prudential aspect of persons in society which depends on the ethical principles or notions as we believe is the other way round for the prudence of health care takers depend on their perception of biological-medical notions. The World Health Organization (WHO) has thus stated "health" in terms of "a state of complete physical, mental and social well-being, not merely the absence of disease and infirmity" or what is the "holistic notion of health", which is crucial in our interactions with the world of medical prudence, and this is not an ethical thesis *per se*. "Why should then we bother about the ethical as separately from the biological?" is the question. In fact, Stahl thinks that if the redundancy is not shown, we would hopelessly confuse the biological for the ethical, the prudential for the moral, which is not welcome. Skipping his lengthy analysis of Kant's moral positions, we come to find the crucial assertion about the debatable point here. He says: "we have come full circle, back to the opening senses of bioethics as a redundancy, for we see again that the principle of ethical judgment inescapably involved in the evaluation of biomedical problems, is precisely the principle presupposed in the reconstituting of the prudentially organized world of the biologically grounded individual so as to permit the emerge of persons"[17].

I must be excused to make a sweeping unpleasant remark about the supporters of redundancy view in bioethics. I must say that their conception about ethics as a field of study within philosophy (but not biology), is grossly confused. This is not uncommon to passionate students of ethics as a subsidiary study to biology, medicine, management etc. I have seen non-philosophers, even those who have good reading of ethics to skip through many important tasks of ethics, which constitutes its nature. *The Primer* (Vol.1) of the Series takes care of this mistake because practical and professional ethics has been thoroughly muddled by misconceptions about ethics itself though we (ethicists) have least confusions about biology and medicine. It may well be that these thinkers trashing biomedical ethics have some confusions about the nature and task of biology and medicine or else, they nourish another confusion, that is, they imagine relation between something like biology and ethics as either synonymous or one of them as redundant (the other being sufficient). We should be first of all clear about relationships, which is not ground of equivalence or synonymy. Let us ask Seedhouse whether he is sure about what is ethics because his "characterization" of "ethics" is *too narrow?* It is too narrow because "ethics" does not merely help us (including doctors) in conducting our life in relation to other human beings in desirable fashion. Ethics does many things; the analysis of the language of ethics, of the justification of ethical norms and most interestingly to answer whether ethicists have any business to deal with questions like value-laden issues in biology and medicine. Seedhouse and Stahl should have realized that their papers fall under "metaethics" and not bioethics or biology because it is about justification of biomedicine as sufficient for any ethical inquiry. However, they must know that metaethics does not depend on biology or medicine. In fact, the logical scrutiny within the field of ethics, which we grossly overlook while "characterizing ethics" is not dependent on biology in anyway. Our position with regard to Wilson must have stressed this point I believe. We also forget that ethics deals with questions of human virtues and values, several psychological factors, and most importantly, resolution of value-laden practical and professional issues, none of which depends exclusively on biology. The last task of ethics is particularly not based on biology by any extent of imagination. This means that biomedical ethics needs clarification of "characterization of ethics" properly before it could be trashed in preference to biomedical science. We shall come to this "characterization" in connection to "relation" among ethics, biology and medicine at a proper place. For now, let us continue with the redundancy argument.

The "claims" of Seedhouse are defect-galore because for one thing, medical ethics has no business about confusing the ethical with the non-ethical and for another thing, it is in no way "parasitic" to normative ethics. In fact, both defects are related because if we have no clear conception about what normative ethics aims at and in what ways practical and professional ethics are relative to ethical normativism. If we do not understand these things well, we shall fall in the trap of calling biomedical ethics as parasitic to ethics or norms of ethics as tool of resolving ethical crises. But why the norms should be thought as means for resolving biomedical problems by interested parties is not understandable. Do norms lose significance if biologists, medical men and ethicists do not take them as tools to mend problems of said sciences? Not at all because norms are not and perhaps cannot be applied in these ways by such and such groups. I said while considering the debate regarding Wilson that there is little doubt about moral agents themselves being biological, that they live in biological environment, interact with beings of different kinds, they gather important moral experiences and knowledge owing to such interactive life with beings and things but that does not prove that ethics depends on man being biological, what to speak of biology. It may be that our ethical ways of thinking and living in society are influenced by our being parts of nature or biotic community but that too does not prove that our being ethical depends on our being biological or that ethics depends on biology. This is so because by virtue of moral knowledge in nature, one is not called ethical or does not become so; the judgment of ethicality depends largely on our corroboration of ethical knowledge and decision-making with other people in a complex situation of prudence and practicality. I believe that our being ethical does not depend on any traditional moral theory either because normative artificiality is refused by collective ethical discourses. If this be the case then biomedical ethics can never be handmaid of normativism because our ethical concerns about the biological and the medical matters themselves remain non-moral, which is not changed by adding "ethics" for signifying "ethical interests" or "ethical concerns" or "ethical scrutiny" in anyway. Biomedicine was, is and will be the same *non-normative factual discipline* for its basic interest is factual and not ethical. Similarly, biomedical ethics is not a new species of biology and medicine; it is though a *species of ethics* as an ever growing field of study within philosophy. Ethics has included many such things from its inception. Perhaps our ethical discoveries or enthusiasm at the present time with discipline like biomedicine is only posterior to theoretical ethics and theoretical biomedicine because ethics *per se* is practical, not merely theoretical jugglery with normative theories or biomedical theories. It does take deep interest in finding out which problems raise questions of ethical desirability, good and just and thus do not remain isolated for the sciences for such study. Ethics shows interests in analyzing and resolving these factual problems which are *value-laden* because modern man should not live with them, and biomedicine is not fully equipped to do the job alone. Hence, for doing this job, we need biomedical ethics, this is to say, biomedical ethics is needed for discovery, analysis and practical resolution of biomedical value-laden issues where traditional norms of ethics are not applied by either ethicists or medical men. This point takes us closer to an understanding of the nature of ethics including practical and professional ethics. I think at this point we should remark that biomedical ethics is species of ethics not because value-resolutions are taken up but also because metaethical and other important ethical concerns mentioned by me are considered. It is interesting to analyze that being truly a branch of ethics proper biomedical ethics has a metaethical task as well. No doubt the aspect of resolution will further reveal that biomedical ethics relies heavily on the sciences of biology and medicine for without critical understanding of the scientific issues, proper ethical appreciation and resolution are impossible. This must prove the close "relation" of biology, medicine and ethics as such but that does not prove that biology, medicine and ethics are all the same or that one is sufficient and others are redundant. Truly, biotechnology shows us that biology may depend on technology or technology on biology in some sense, that is, they are deeply related but does that prove that biotechnology is redundant or that either biology or technology is sufficient or that both are similar or synonymous. Biomedicine as an independent discipline does not constitute biomedical ethics, whereas biomedical ethics as an independent study within ethics is not within biomedicine. Seedhouse does not have any apathy (it appears) to accept that ethics is sufficient to constitute biomedical ethics, which however will not be liked by Wilson and others. What Seedhouse fails to recognize is that his 'ethical A' is valuable in so far as it is a body of normative theories having direct relevance to 'ethical B', wherein we care much for active work like those of health care professionals. This is a great mistake because 'ethical B' does not need 'ethical A' at all if that means taking the "right tool from tool-box to mend professional ethical problems" (see vol. 1). Seedhouse has written so much about ethics education in medicine, Cassell must be aware of it but why didn't they care about the simple fact that for professionals in health care it is neither necessary nor sufficient to be educated about traditional normative theories in ethics is strange enough. Why were they worried about the way Kant may be applied to solve the value-laden problem of euthanasia or Sartre's existential ethical thesis be applied to mend suicide? This is because many non-ethicists have the confusion that if we do not apply theories, what on earth is application of ethics and for that matter biomedical ethics is not known to us. If we have vagueness about biomedical ethics as this one, that is, we are not sure if it has relation to application of ethics, how can we be sure about what exactly biomedical ethics is? Much confusion, therefore, is about the nature and tasks of biomedical ethics which we are trying to clarify here. Let us clarify now that even if biomedical ethics does not apply one or many ethical theories for being ethically oriented as health professionals, still biomedical ethics makes great sense – it is still extremely practical in another way. Seedhouse and others must be convinced that biomedical ethics is not handmaid of normativism and ethical engineering (see vol.1), and, therefore, not redundant rather sensibly independent within the broad field of ethics (and not biology). These thinkers must be convinced now that an ethical venture in the realm of factual sciences like this one, makes it under ethics and not under the sciences because *per se* the sciences do not consider performing such task, whereas ethics does consider performing such tasks. Ethics is essentially interdisciplinary when it is "practical", and being closer to our occupations and professions, but it does not undermine the value of the sciences and other fields where it is applied to resolve value-laden issues.

The ground is ripe for us to remind Dr. Cassell that even if Seedhouse were silent or neutral about which ethical norm to apply for 'ethical B', it was a welcome move on the part of Seedhouse because he must have realized the problems of choosing one among many theories all appearing to be very fruitful but turns out to be not so fruitful when 'ethical B' becomes vital for doctors or nurses. Does Cassell suffer from the same confusion that biomedical ethics must be theory-dependent? If she has such idea, she cannot be against Seedhouse's "Against thesis". Her inclination for artificiality in applying norms comes out clearly when she is very sorry about Seedhouse leaving out Kantianism. And she is annoyed when Seedhouse appears to be "naturalistic". Now, this "naturalism" has pleased and displeased many of us in ethics. We are pleased because it has some substance with regard to logical definitions and logical derivations in ethics but we are displeased when every naturalist is seen as ill-fated for committing the 'naturalistic fallacy'. Truly, Seedhouse's view that biomedical ethics is redundant because 'ethical A' is predominant has many flaws but I have not found a "naturalistic fallacy" being committed by Seedhouse in his thesis. Frankena has well taught us that being overenthusiastic about finding this fallacy where there is none is itself a fallacy. I have argued in Vol. 1 that every naturalist need not commit this fallacy, at least not J.S. Mill in *Utilitarianism*. Seedhouse never says that ethical "good" ought to be logically defined or that 'ethical B' should be logically derived from 'ethical A'. What he says is that for the factual sciences it may not be possible to independently construct what is ethically desirable for health care takers. Is this a case of naturalistic fallacy even if Seedhouse is a naturalist? Is there distant logical relation between 'being a naturalist' and 'committing naturalistic fallacy'? I do not think that Cassell is right in charging ontological and epistemological inconsistencies in Seedhouse's views because he does not aim at any ontological thesis at all by saying that ethics is the basis of biology and medicine and is not like Wilson or others who did have an ontological thesis. For Seedhouse it was perfectly consistent to maintain that normative ethics is different from biology and medicine and *necessary* for ethical considerations in biology and medicine. However, he was grossly inconsistent to conclude that, therefore, biomedical ethics is non-existent, we do not need it. I think, if he said that ethics is sufficient for all ethical considerations in biology and medicine, he would be equally inconsistent. Why on earth in biomedical ethics we do not need both the factual and the ethical, is not known to me. Cassell should be reminded that in upholding the case of biomedical ethics by criticizing views like Wilson and Seedhouse, clear statement of tasks of ethics is needed. It is also important to demonstrate that biomedical ethics is within ethics, it is closely related to biology and medicine and may be justified as an independent branch of ethics.

After a lengthy talk about Seedhouse and Cassell, considering the case of Štahl may be easy because we have seen the problems in maintaining "ontological" thesis that ethics is derived from biology and the "judgmental" thesis that biomedical issues and ethical issues are non-distinguishable. We contest Stahl's point that many so-called biological issues may be reduced to the factual or the non-ethical because even if the meaning clarification of the notions of "person", "life", "death", "health" are all not mere play of words but factually (scientifically) grounded, equally true is that ethical concerns about "life", "death" and "health" are not resolved merely by language-games and scientific scrutiny but by systematic ethical effort, called the practical effort of the professional life. What things are proved if we know qua physicians that "person" is this and not that when after such knowledge we do not ask how to tame the raging ethical disagreements among professionals about desirability of making or taking life in our civil societies? There is no doubt that ethical care about making and taking life will naturally fall in turmoil of ethical debates, where *meaning* of life (the factually given) should be crucial though not necessarily be the only aid to find a way out of the turmoil. Stahl should know that in practical and professional ethics we cannot go for eternity in isolation or association for arm-chair churnings, it needs dynamics on our part and it transcends subjectivism of all kinds, including the fallacy of mere analysis of meaning of concepts by intellectuals. Hence, any chauvinist idea of biomedical science as sufficient or ontologically basic is as defective as ethics is sufficient or ontologically basic. Why has this peculiar idea of "this is basic to that" come in such matters? Perhaps, non-philosophers can't digest intrusions by philosophers or, philosophers as they are habitually fault finders, cannot accept the naturalists. It is bad habit though to believe that "ethics is our business – no entry for outsiders".

All this now takes us to the justification of biomedical ethics (in no less unambiguous terms, I said). Well, I have been considering this task seriously while I was analyzing the strengths and weaknesses in redundancy thesis. I should be more clear and specific now. Readers are aware by this time that "ethics" should not be scrappily understood. A fairly complete statement of its task leads us to realize that it is a branch of philosophy dealing with the normative, the metaethical and the practical tasks. In addition to these we deal with psychological basis of ethics, virtues and values, professional and occupational value-laden issues and their resolution and value concerns in ecological matters. Interestingly, our tasks do not include ethical concerns in biomedical, educational, economic, business, management, social and political matters but we know that all these are well within the purview of ethics as we understand it now and not within economics, management and so on. There is no point left for us to argue that "managerial ethics" is redundant as management studies are fundamental and sufficient. According to me, therefore, when we are speaking about "ethics" as a subject, we should find out whether any species within its realm carries at least some of the major tasks of "ethics". To "justify" that biomedical ethics as "ethical discussions pertain to biomedicine" and nothing more or nothing less, should "justify" that *issues* within biomedicine truly pertains to ethical study and that study itself bears some properties of the genus "ethics". Let us come to the latter part first. Biomedical ethics takes up some *metaethical* task about which I have said something before. To be precise, my relentless effort of "justification" of biomedical ethics within ethics and not redundant therefore is to perform a *metaethical* task under biomedical ethics. In fact, perhaps unknowingly, Wilson, Seedhouse and even Stahl were performing the said 'metaethical task' though their findings were not as our findings. Wilson and Seedhouse's efforts of negative justification were well within biomedical ethics as I believe. Or, were they discussing biology and/or medicine? *Socio-biology* of Wilson or another book of the supporter of the redundancy arguments are better treated as works dealing with biomedical ethics and not biology or medicine. Hence, biomedical ethics could not be trashed; it remains perhaps more strongly within ethics because its immunity system is stronger now. The negative justifications to trash biological ethics have strengthened its immunity system. Strangely, analysis of "biomedical ethics", every part of it in fact for *clarification of meaning* is another metaethical task, which some people wrongly took as either pure biological and medical discussion or pure ethical discussion based on biology. The matter is again not of any confusion because clarity of reason and systemization of aids to clarify meaning of basic notions in biomedical ethics is the focus of our attention, which is metaethical focus and nothing else. We shall shortly find out that application of traditional ethical norms as either useful or not useful is another metaethical task in biomedical ethics, which leads to consider the justifiable *model of application of ethics* in the field of biomedicine. This way careful reader might find other metaethical tasks of biomedical ethics. I must say that logic of relation among philosophy, biology, medicine and ethics makes a good case for metaethical study when biomedicine is taken as a study not disjoint from philosophy and ethics.

When we come to the normative task and practical or applied task, the participation of biomedical ethics is even clearer. *Traditionally* biomedical ethics has the habit (bad!) of discussing some established ethical norms like Kantian deontology, Mill's utilitarianism, existential ethics, Thomism etc. and then finding out which theory fits where as if a definite nut should fit a fixed bolt. It is undeniable that biomedical ethics is concerned about the value of normative ethics with regard to the value-laden issues like abortion, euthanasia and so on. Better habit must be to find out how such theories or others were *found to be effective in the real dynamics of resolution of value-laden issues* in biomedical field but that takes us to the nature and model of application of ethics and practical ethics. Yet, we should not forget that being completely unaware of standard norms is not a good habit either because finding out the practical value of norms in value-resolutions call for awareness of normative ethics. It is clear that traditionally biomedical ethics has been wrongly understood as artificial application of ethical norms like Kantianism to find out how it leads to resolve euthanasia or In Vitro experiments, which may not be taken as the proper model of application of ethics in biomedical cases. In my mind (stated already in vols. 1 and 2), application of ethics is not application of standard norms in such cases by ethicists or biologists or physicians, rather, it is a joint effort of all concerned parties in our societies who participate in moral dialogues to reach consensus about such value-laden issues for effective resolution and decision-making rules, which are matters of constant debates. This model of application, which I have called "intersubjective corroboration", speaks about defects in ethical engineering with norms by all power assuming ethicists and bio-scientists. If we take this to be true, the discovery of effective theories is only posterior to ethical application. We have ample evidences in contemporary application of ethics wherein this or something close to it has helped societies to find out ways out of biomedical ethical impasse. That this is not a blank talk shall be revealed in some of the chapters to follow. For now, we stress on biomedical ethics as performing the applied task as most important because why on earth should value-laden issues be simply discovered by wise people rather than not solving them? Biomedical ethics is well within ethics as it is concerned with finding out human virtues and values rather than principles as effective in resolving biomedical ethical impasse. Much talk about this can be traced in "anti-principlism" and "virtue based ethics" in recent times.

Most important it is to notice that we talk sensitively about occupational, sub-professional and professional ethics within ethics (see Vol. 1) because in several occupations like engineering or business, in sub-professions like nursing and in professions like medical profession or teaching, many value-laden issues emerge for resolution. A civil society cannot leave them on fate because we have realized that some stark-factual issues are never solved and accepted amicably among people when they are resolved by professionals of a field, though there is much hue and cry about professionals being best parties to do such things. Whereas others believe that professionals need ethicists and many other parties of relevance for such things to do. Again this is a matter of justifying models in professional ethics. What is most important here is to notice that professional bio-scientists and medical men, sub-professionals in the entire health care system and other professionals like political decision-makers and those involved in the distribution of health care services to people should discuss abut ethical matters pertaining to health care. This is clear evidence that when we consider the broad field of professional, occupational and sub-professional ethics, biomedical ethics comes in relation to all these fields. I have reservations to say that ethical concerns in biology and medicine are merely within professional ethics because it has deep relations with practical ethics (the sense in which I take it) and with occupational, sub-professional and even with environmental ethics.

As we stand now, biomedical ethics is not a species of biology or medicine. Ethics on the other hand, does happily engage itself in many cases of biology and medicine and there is no point in justifying its redundancy. We should realize by now that why I am so opposed to the idea of Cassell, Seedhouse and Stahl that ethics is predominantly normative and for that reason their thesis that biomedicine being scientific in nature, ethics has no role to play in it or that there is nothing such as biomedical ethics. It is ethics with which we are dealing now, and within it, bioethics cannot be downplayed as pathology cannot be downplayed being within the broader biological science. In the next chapter we will further consider some more problems in biomedical ethics.

NOTES

1. Mahowald, Mary B., "Biomedical Ethics: A Precocious Youth" in Joseph P. De Macro and R.M. Fox (eds.), *New Directions in Ethics: The Challenge*

of Applied Ethics, Routledge and Kegan Paul, NY, pp. 144-45.
2. Singer, Peter, *The Expanding Circle*, OUP, Oxford, 1981, p. 55.
3. *Ibid*, p. 71.
4. *Ibid*, p. 72.
5. *Ibid*, p. 77.
6. *Ibid*, p. 84.
7. *Ibid*, p. 85.
8. *Ibid*, p. 147.
9. Seedhouse, D.F., "Against medical ethics: a philosopher's view", *Medical Education*, Vol. 25, 1991, pp. 280-82.
10. Readers may refer to D.F. Seedhouse's works: *Health: the foundation for achievement*, John Wiley, 1986; *Ethics: the heart of health care*, John Wiley, 1988; *Liberating medicine*, John Wiley, 1972; *Fortress NHS: a philosophical review of the National Health Service*, John Wiley, 1994; *Reforming health care: the philosophy and practice of international health reform*, John Wiley, 1995 and *Health promotion: philosophy, prejudice and practice*, John Wiley, 1997.
11. Seedhouse, D.F., "Against medical ethics: a philosophical view", *op. cit.*, p. 280.
12. Seedhouse, D.F., "Against medical ethics: a response to Cassell", *British Medical Journal*, Vol. 24, 1998, p. 13.
13. *Ibid*, p. 15.
14. Stahl, Gary, "Bioethics: A Redundant Concept" in E. Morscher and R. Stranzinger (eds.), *Ethics: Foundation, problems and applications* Kluwer, London, 1998.
15. *Ibid*, p. 285.
16. *Ibid*, p. 285.
17. *Ibid*, p. 297.

2

Some More Problems in Biomedical Ethics

I start this chapter not abruptly as it appears from its title because reference to "some more problems" in biomedical ethics here is in fact in addition to some problems we have already discussed. There is no wonder that in the first chapter (Nature and Justification of Biomedical Ethics) we were considering "some problems" truly speaking because we tried our best to clarify our position with regard to several confusions about and attacks on biomedical ethics. The problem simply stated is: Is biomedical ethics possible within ethics? We believe that our clarification unambiguously answered the problem in the affirmative. In doing so it has also clarified the meaning of "bio", "medical" and "biomedical" along with "ethics" and "biomedical ethics", which amounts to a proper understanding of what "biomedical ethics" consists in or what is its "nature". We have also argued that clarification of "nature" of biomedical ethics is inseparably related to the problem of "justification" of ethical talk in the fields of biology and medicine because if we do not know the real significance of "biomedical ethics" there is hardly any point in justifying the case of such ethics. Equally true is that if we do not have enough reasons (not necessarily strict logical arguments) to justify that ethics, as a branch of philosophy, performing the important tasks it has, should undertake the task of ethical scrutiny of some practical problems emerging in biology and medicine, it is pointless to project biomedical ethics as having such and such features or characteristics. The initial or the starting problems enthusiastically raised by sceptics to show inadequacies in such interdisciplinary ventures were therefore faced with some success as we believe it, we still have "some more problems" to be considered further so that residual vagueness about biomedical ethics is eradicated.

To my mind we may now consider three more problems regarding this matter: (A) what do we mean by *value-laden practical problems* in the field of biomedicine and how best should these problems be *categorized for analysis and resolution?* (B) how should such problems be *resolved?* And (C), are ethical norms and principles basic to resolution of these problems or do we have any other *model of ethical resolution?* The first problem, related closely to the sceptical problem discussed earlier, asks about the sense in which practical problems may be sensibly called "value-laden", and if we have such problems, how to enlist them for they may be many as well as overlapping. The second problem is about methodology of resolving these problems which is again related to the problems of accepting normativism or principlism and ethical engineering therein. We may then come to the last inquiry about the justified "model" of resolving value-laden biological problems. Resolving these problems (some more) is extremely important for us as not having a clear idea about the range of biomedical ethical problems and ways to arrange them under broad groups, our next task to resolve them might be highly unsystematic and often beyond practical management. This will also help us in our theoretical effort to analyze several problems more conveniently according to their family resemblance within a group amounting to fewer intricacies in nitty-gritty of the pragmatics involved in the real life encountering and resolution of these problems. The problem of adequate 'methodology' in ethical resolution of biomedical problems is needed for subjective ways or unmethodical ways in such matters are like encouraging quacks in medicine. We should know how ethics ought to be applied when it comes to resolution of matters of far reaching social consequences. In this regard, unavoidable questions of adequacy of applying standard ethical theories and principles in order to resolve bioethical crisis comes to our mind and there are strong sceptical grounds to reject both normativism and principlism. This might be possible if we justify finally the way or method to move beyond ethical engineering with norms and principles. Let us take up these problems now.

Coming first to the value-laden or ethical problems in biology and medicine and their classification or listing according to family resemblance, I must say that all practical problems emerging constantly in the fields of biology and medicine are found to be 'value-laden' or raising ethical questions of right, good, just and desirable etc. not by subjective perception. Hence, ethicists or health care experts by virtue of their theoretical and practical wisdom cannot and should not put moral value to an issue because more often than not personal value imputations are either obsessed by chauvinistic ideas or they are simply outbursts of blind emotions. In many cases imputation of value from outside by a person carries little or no social or public recognition. Such things are also found against people's perception as well as people's welfare. This is not to say that an ethicist or a physician or other interested parties are not able to discover a practical problem as value-laden or that they need not contribute to the discovery of such things, but "discovery" as I say now, is quite different from "putting a value" to a problem. It is one thing to 'discover' in the milieu of public life and interactive public affairs that such and such practical problems are not stark factual ones pertaining to "what is" rather pertains to "what ought to be" or "what should be the case" and it is another thing to apply our whims or emotions to stress that such and such problems must be taken as ethical problems in public life and public affairs. When I speak of 'public life' and 'public affairs' I do not have any idea to exclude the groups of health caretakers, the physicians, the nurses and others. However, I will not simply put much stress on these groups responsible for "discovering" value-laden problems because the intricate "discovery" (if we really feel the intricacy), is close to a collective in which the health caretakers are inseparably bound to their clients (if that is a proper term to use), that is, to whom they are bound by some duties, responsibilities and obligations. And these people though having little or no idea about stark biomedical problems have the 'moral authority' to participate in finding out the questions of value imminent in these problems because they are the ones who suffer the brunt of such problems in our societies. Equally true is that our health caretakers suffer the brunt of these problems as well for it is they who face them for immediate resolution to come out of moral dilemma and to come out in flying colours in face of duties, responsibilities and obligations they have, not for any gain or fear or pride necessarily. We need not forget that many health caretakers though aware of the value-ladenness of the practical problems have little regard for them, that is, care least for discovery of what should be done and in what ways. In fact, the discovery of ethical problems is itself a public affair, health caretakers being party to these problems. Such discoveries appear to be almost instantaneous as if some queer intention helps us to do so but without falling back to such queer things, one may reasonably speak about the moral experiences and knowledge one has about ought and should of practical problems by virtue of a participant in this complex life we live among many beings and things. It does not therefore need a deep knowledge of In Vitro and In Utero experiments for ordinary people or sound knowledge of the theory and practice of abortion to discover that such issues are not merely problematic for our physicians and nurses but largely for the individuals who are often looked upon as "subjects" of such experiments and procedures, as well as for those who are conscious social people in civil societies – the lawyers, the businessmen who run a nursing home for instance, where such things are done and even the government and non-government agencies who are directly or indirectly responsible for connecting themselves to these issues as parts of social responsibility and not to remain aloof. Hence, any practical problem that is value-laden or those having ethical import are not so by the effort of either professional ethicists or professional doctors. Even the "discovery" or "knowledge" of these value-laden problems is not only owing to the professional enterprises of ethicists and physicians, a large body of the public does help us in realizing that several problems raise questions of ethical value and need resolution. A good instance may be the realization of euthanasia as a practical problem in the field of medicine which is also 'value-laden' because the truth is evident to a doctor or a nurse once they come in association to the patient in helpless condition, the close associates of the patient and a number of lawyers and the public who express positive or negative reactions, mostly as I believe on ethical-pragmatic grounds. It is not difficult to find some typical reactions of physicians and nurses who think that euthanasia for them is not worth considering as an ethically charged practical problem because for them it is a matter of pragmatics, prudence and rational decision-making having no relation whatsoever with what some people think about its ethical significance. In fact, for these people, the doctors and the nurses, treating a person in a vegetative condition should decide whether or not his or her request for ending life should be medically allowed and if so, the way it needs to be done not for any moral reasons but for the ground realities of existence – the practical ones so to say. Now, if we allow these people having no care for the "discovery" of the value-laden aspect of the issue, and allow them to do what their prudence sanctions, every other person wanting medically associated death, should have what they want. Or, may be in any case their prudence does not sanction any such things even if enough moral grounds are there for such medical intervention. In both cases, a disturbing question remains unanswered: 'why at all euthanasia is or is not desirable or good?' Answer to this question enables our sceptical physicians and nurses to realize that based on the ground realities of existence, need or no-need of euthanasia may not be justified at all because more often than not the answers go beyond these practical, pragmatic and prudential aspects to hit the aspects of good, just, right, obligatory, responsible, duty on the part of the deciders to take one's life just because one allows it to end or the others believe that doing so is pragmatic. Well, the ground reality may be understandable; the sick person is in a terrible state, his or her physical-mental condition unbearable, the family have run out of all resources and are at the verge of break-down condition, still the question (terribly nagging one) disturbs us, 'is it still desirable to take life?' Equally important ground reality may be that the sick person has been forced to give a statement or has been psychologically frustrated or systematically neglected or planned by the crooked to grab his or her wealth, still the nagging question remains, 'what should be done?' Should we take life? In such cases we find that falling prey to the clumsy nitty-gritty of ground realities would be tying one knot after another than opening them unless a serious effort has been made to transcend such questions by asking more basic one: 'why at all is it *ethically permissible* to take one's life while the given stark facts are that someone wants it and other do not for such and such practical reasons?' So the wise doctor's judgment that 'vegetable should die now' or the harried patient's judgment that 'I am fed up, help me please' or for some cunning: 'for him, all cannot die' may not be good grounds to take life at all. It is the collective mind, the thinking and deciding public who has to decide on such matters, that becomes a law if needed. The question of "taking life", therefore, is not merely a subjective decision on practical grounds; it needs something more, scrutinizing the questions of desirability or ethicality so to say, which leads us to know why taking life is an ethical-practical affair or unethical and impractical affair despite the prevailing laws of societies which may or may not allow it at the present time on different practical grounds. Truly speaking, discovery of the "moral" in the "practical" and the "legal" is often responsible in transcending the hackneyed "practical" and the "legal" to give them a new face, a humane face most of the time.

A physician, a nurse, a sick person and others who have care for discovery of such things can come together to find that "taking life" is not an easy affair after all. Let us not forget that there are physicians, nurses, sick people and others who believe that human life is very precious for different reasons and it would be extremely undesirable to "take" it medically. Any disregard shown to such people by our said stern-faced prudential persons is a kind of chauvinism, which our modern world does not like so much. In medicine, "I am the boss" does not matter much as in ethics, there are no bosses.

Much has been said about the "knowledge" or "discovery" of biomedical problems as "ethically charged" but we have to be more elaborate about the exact "methodology" of such discovery by all concerned parties though some hint has been given on our behalf about the *participation of the public* in such a discovery because matters raising ethical questions is a matter of realization in this active public life. Ethically charged matters being social, cannot transcend social beings. It is important to read what G.H. Kieffer has to say in his essay on "Ethical Decision-Making" in his work *Bioethics* (1979): "The recognition of an ethical problem is not always easy. To be effective, *ethical methodology* (my italics) requires that the identification of the problem be as clear as possible in order to reduce uncertainty and ambiguity".[1] The *identification* of the problem (for me "discovery"), says Kieffer, is difficult but not impossible if we follow a proper method. Much like what we have found, Kieffer says, "Whether our social structure can withstand the strain of haphazard application when fundamental values are meddled with is very much an issue. The current abortion issue bears testimony to the discrepancy between what is being done and what ought to be done. Our society lacks a *moral consensus* (my italics)[2] from which we may draw". Clearly, discovery of morally charged problems in biomedical science needs some sort of dealing with the collective consensus. Kieffer goes on, much to our liking again: "Depending on *experts* (my italics)[3] – whether they are physicians, scientists, moralists or theologians – is no solution either... Even within the context of a single religion (e.g. Christianity), directives are sufficiently vague as to be subject to quite different interpretation". Truly, finding out value-laden problems rules out ethical chauvinism by ethicists and physicians. Equally true is that ethical pluralism as a way to reach selection of values, cannot be valid either.

I would like to state the "methodology" of recognition of value-laden biomedical problems in the following steps:

1. Listen, read and think about a practical statement which is problematic in the field of biomedical science carefully (if needed, repeatedly), to have a first hand idea of the involvement of the element of ethical "ought" in practical "is".
2. For this there is no need for any participating party in the vast social milieu to read academic ethics or to go to a sophistical ethics *guru* for guidance.
3. Rather, there is need to be open minded and respecting towards what professionals and non-professionals think and say about the said statement.
4. But there is no need to be so blindly respecting as to grant any one view to be absolutely true. We should better concentrate on disagreements and agreements about such matters.
5. Most important is to find in this context the grounds based on which the debating people transcend the practical aspects of a problem to concentrate on aspects of desirability, good, just, right, duty, obligation and responsibility qua social people.
6. The value charged practical questions thus found in biomedicine should not be further analyzed theoretically until practical ways to resolve them are obtained, needing fresh set of methods to do such things.

An analysis of these steps, which are not mechanical or artificial rather suggestive cues to "discovery" and for that reason, may be continuously revised for betterment, first calls our non-chauvinist, declassed, learning mind *qua* professionals rather than a bossing attitude or 'only I know such things' attitude, or else, not even a step is put forward. This has been more explicitly stated in 2, 3 and 4 after the first hand idea of what a value-laden practical problem could be like (as in 1). Though step 1 is initial in all respects because without experiencing an assertion in the social context like "medical termination of life *should be* allowed", there is no point in searching for "ought" element in what "is". It is important here to notice that being attracted to further ethical scrutiny of such matters is not exclusive to a physician or a nurse, it is open to anyone lest the person is interested in not only getting wiser or is a sufferer whose associate has met termination of life rather wants to move further for an active participation in the resolution of the matter. There is no greatness as I think to get enthusiastic about writing pages full of intellectual brightness what it means to medically terminate life, fill our audience with flowering words of wisdom and to show what he or she believes to be true rather, it is important to go forward to resolution of such problems in association with other people. There is nothing worth in step 1 therefore if all is read and known but not done for resolution. This is of course a matter of training and temperament to find some interest in such matters but academics help only in limited way when it comes to "take some social interest". The seriously interested people in step 1 thus get an idea about the fact that some assertions pertaining to the field of biology and medicine do not merely close door on common people and other concerned parties because such problems are not merely about what the medical fraternity thinks to be best is in fact the best, rather what the medical fraternity and we too, *should* do. The crux of the interest is that such assertions are not simplistic but extremely problematic; as they challenge us for a moral debate, there is no easy cut and dried way to instantly face them and solve them as required doses of antibiotics are used for treating specific ailments. However, physicians know very well that some doses of vitamins given to a nagging wealthy person who has gone maniac over loss of a pound does call for some question for "ought"; such cases are not simplistic. Many government decisions therefore call for serious public ethical scrutiny for doses of irons and vitamins to the poor Indian girl child and women call for some debate as doses of balanced diet or some diet recommendable for healthy living at least may be more pressing a need than iron pills and vitamins. Do irons and vitamins work when women live on mango seeds? More interesting is for us now, do we leave this question as practical or does it not call for the discovery of a debate about immersed "ought" in a stark "is"? There is all likelihood of a legal statement regarding medical affairs pressed on us for such moral discovery. There must be some reason I believe to declare early law as redundant to embrace a new one regarding euthanasia in the Netherlands. In fact biomedical laws change and grow not from anything but from serious moral churning. Hence, step 1 is as important as a starter in the "method" of moral discovery in biomedical matters.

Closely associated to 'de-classism' in ethical discovery is the careful avoidance of theory co-option by the interested parties because ethical readings do not make us any wiser by a fraction or the association of an ethics *guru* does not make us any noble. This is so because ethics as such most likely do not ever attempt to make us ethical as logical rules are not aimed at making us logical though ethical knowledge we have is potent to be useful in public life to resolve moral crises as knowing rules of logic is useful in analysis of intricate theses. Hence, our first idea about moral value in a biomedical problem does not call upon us to start reading ethics so that we become more and more ethically charged or ethically able to discover the questions of ought. Non-ethicists such as many physicians are, have uncanny ability to smell the same ought as ethicists do or may be very ordinary man, a "lay person" in medical term knows the "ought" without ethical and medical knowledge. In fact, theory non-cooption is welcome than theory cooption because ethical knowledge of theories might govern us in a patterned way than having an open mind. There is nothing great in thinking first hand without much analysis that the problem of euthanasia is a moral problem *because* "life is intrinsically good" and we have to perform our "duty" *qua* human beings to "respect" the "inherently valuable". Even if you teach such great thesis to someone, biomedical problems having ethical overtones might be perceived differently as another one among us might have totally different set of reasons though he or she may not have any idea about deontology, teleology and so on. Recognizing the value-ladenness of euthanasia needs enthusiastic mixing, debating, talking, reading or to say remaining "open" to social life and social affairs from where we draw the nectar of moral knowledge and thus the knowledge of hovering "ought" in practical "is". Intellectuals of high class fail to realize the same in isolation therefore; they often tend to be set-minds, ever boastful of their wisdom. This truth has been stated in step 3 of our "method" where de-classed professionals and non-professionals have been urged to stay catholic in the face of theoretic and intellectual bigotry in biomedicine. However, it has been further urged in step 4 that it is undesirable to forget what one thinks, analyses and knows than blindly following one view or the other of professionals or non-professionals regarding this matter. It would be extremely poor on our part to imagine us less educated or not having ethical or medical background to not to discover what we should because we may turn out to be extremely contributing to the field of biomedicine by virtue of our plain thoughts and deeds. In fact, moral debates which portray moral agreements and disagreements are again not exclusive affairs of intellectuals. We know by this time that the value problem in abortion is a serious one. Its resolution is pressing enough because the aborted or likely to be aborted or wanting to be aborted women, those women who oppose abortion and others who ponder over pros and cons of the same do ask for the resolution of the value-laden moral issue called "abortion". More often than not our efforts to resolve such problems are helped by belligerent moral views. Hence, finding a problem as value-laden is an intricate affair of remaining "open" to the social milieu or precisely to the *social experiences* we have. With this comes the idea that for finding out value questions in practical affairs we do not need *a priori* thinking or intuitive faculties, it is a plain matter of having complex social experiences.

This last point is extremely important, which has been stated more clearly in step 5 because remaining "open" (or as wise men say, keep your cognitive faculties open), is closely related to knowing what people think about the value aspects of abortion even though they do not know much about the practical aspects of abortion. This is to say that we should remain open to transcend the academic complexities of abortion to filter out the different grounds on which the act has been justified as good or bad, right or wrong, and desirable and undesirable. To be precise, moral brooding on practical affairs is to be more focused as here our concern is exactly that. However, it would be a grave error to avoid some important practical aspects of abortion or even the academic part because without having any idea about the real life cases of abortion, the emergency of doing so or the necessity part of the termination, we should not jump to any conclusion. It is exactly due to this that remaining open to biomedical matters does not rule out knowing from our physicians and nurses about what they do or have to do and most importantly, why they think they should do or they must do when cases come knocking at their doors. Reasonable is to believe that discovery of value-laden practical problems in biomedicine is truly a social affair, physicians and technical persons being no less social, are parties to it. This takes us to the final step (No. 6) which is perhaps the first step to application of ethics at the social level because resolution of the filtered out ethically charged biomedical problems are most important, but that is a different story to which we shall come shortly. For now, let me say that the discovery of bioethical questions is not passionate effort of ethicists, physicians and others because that is something "interesting". Nothing is so "interesting" if that thing is merely peeled layer by layer for deeper theoretical churning, rather it becomes interesting when real life "resolution" is at stake. It is a matter of simple understanding that biomedical ethics is not a handmaid of intellectual passion; it is rather needed for our *discovery and resolution* of morally charged problems emerging in the field of biology and medicine. If we forget this, discovering a problem and arm-chair theoretic churnings are not only useless, they are anti-social attitudes. Members of a civil society need to move on to peoples' ethics, another milestone to non-chauvinism in biomedical ethics about which the rest of the book is all about.

There is another problem in biomedical ethics emerging now as we have stressed on the importance of "resolution" of value-laden biomedical problems rather than sitting pretty well on theoretical analysis. The emerging problem is what are these "ethically charged problems" filtered by concerned people through social interaction in the process of germination and flourishing of biomedical ethics? This is, in fact, the problem of *enlisting and grouping* the manifold bioethical problems which have evolved through a long time in our times. We consider this task as very important, knowing fully well that biology and medicine is growing rapidly and one wonders where it would give up! Naturally, therefore, it is not an exaggeration to say that the era of biology and medicine is one of considering several value-laden problems for resolution. Nevertheless, a number of important things for our perusal soon make us a confused lot if we do not know the systematic way to approach these problems or issues. We cannot really hope to go through the intricacies of all these problems as they appear now for analysis and resolution so easily but we have one good way to at least group some problems for their "family resemblance", that is, their affinity to a basic or crucial ethical question though independently the instances within the groups are marked by their own characteristics and nuances. It is not difficult to resolve these problems when they are grouped because several moral questions regarding these problems are closely related. Yet, when it comes to a closer resolution amounting to concrete formulation of decision-making rules or codes, we have to approach each problem separately with the concerned parties in moral resolution. Equally important is to notice that the theoretical-practical aspect of each problem within a group needs clarification in unambiguous terms so that their effects on moral scrutiny and decision-making could be noticed clearly. It is over-simplistic, therefore, to say that though abortion, euthanasia and assisted suicide bear 'family resemblance' and should be put under one group of value-laden biomedical problem for analysis and resolution, it will be enough to know about one problem to know about the theoretical-practical complexities of the other and thus resolution to one problem leads to the resolution of other problems. Let us remember that in moral matters as present in practical cases, we have a bad habit to skip through many important aspects. There is no doubt therefore that we should consider each value-laden problem on its merit but here our point is whether or not we have some good way to consider the moral questions emerging within a group without skimping.

I am very sorry however to notice that much importance has been given to the standard ethical theories or norms and principles as well as codes and commands in many books on biomedical ethics as if they are necessary, if not sufficient, grounds for a meaningful discourse on the theoretical and the resolution aspects of biomedical ethics. It is not easy to understand why these things should be taken as groundwork to biomedical ethical discussion when we believe that talk about theories and principles comes almost at the end of resolution of biomedical problems. I will come to it at a proper place. For now, I must say that knowledge of norms and principles neither helps us in knowing about value-laden nature of the problems, nor does these things help us in resolution of these problems though they have unique value in so far as they emerge prominently in moral dialogues which is again a matter of "discovery" and not "preoccupation with theories". I must say that the idea of "theory first and then problems for resolution" is a wayward idea. Here we would find that the classification of value charged biomedical problems as per "family resemblance" is also not helped by knowledge of ethical theories and principles because apart from other reasons, one reason is that identifying similar characteristics for grouping of issues is helped by our theoretical and practical knowledge of the biomedical sciences and by our "discovery" of questions of values imminent in these issues. Here one might ask: 'You have said that common people are able to filter out value questions imminent in biomedical issues despite their lack of knowledge of deep theoretical-practical aspects of these issues and now you say that grouping is helped largely by theoretical-practical aspects of these issues. Does it mean that common people do not have the authority of the act of grouping?' The question appears to be a serious one apparently. In reality, the question is a little out of way because we have steadily maintained that people's participation in the resolution of bioethical problems is needed which presupposes their involvement in knowing about the value-laden aspect of such problems, but here we are asking the way a task to be taken up more seriously by the health care professionals and the ethicists in grouping and in the act of corroboration of moral dialogues. It will be extremely difficult for lay persons to group value-laden problems as per their family resemblance or to frame ethical questions for a moral dialogue or to go through nitty-gritty of decision-making rules. However, all these limitations of common people are welcome as something unique is left for the physicians, nurses and ethicists to do in biomedical ethics. Apart from discovery of ethical issues these people are particularly helpful in *grouping of issues*, *framing questions for moral dialogues*, *conduct dialogues*, *analyze them and formulate decision-making rules*. This is not chauvinism against which I was spitting venom because the other concerned parties, the common people have their internal restrictions or limits in the whole affair of biomedical ethics. Hence, accepting the fact that "grouping" of biomedical ethical problems need first hand idea about the theoretical-practical aspects of biomedical sciences, some common ethical experiences and knowledge of academic ethics, we now proceed with a more or less acceptable grouping of such problems.

"Death and Dying" are two pet issues in bioethics. As one goes through a number of works in this field, most of them as I have said earlier, would give an account of ethical theories and principles and then take some value-laden issues like abortion and euthanasia to show the ways in which such issues might be resolved following a theory or a principle or a group of theories and principles. Other authors take a different method of discussion; they would explain a theory or a principle and then show the inherent capacities of these theories and principles to solve such and such value-laden biomedical issues. Avoiding any remark on these methods, here I would draw attention towards an interesting fact. Sampling of works on biomedical ethics reveals that in order to show the applicative aspect of moral theories and principles, these works almost certainly take up the issues related to taking human life, allowing humans to die and even ways to use the dead, i.e., they deal with death and dying roughly with many other issues as well but mostly the cases of death and dying comes up for discussion. No wonder we may find an entire voluminous encyclopaedia on these subjects in the broad field of bioethics. Naturally, therefore, any classification of bioethical issues should take care of at least one broad group wherein cases of human death and dying are included. This I believe is irrespective of the fact that theories and principles have been considered before such grouping for discussion. I strongly believe that though act of classification of bioethical problems is closely related to their resolution or else it is sheer fruitless intellectualism but classification does not necessarily beg *a priori* wisdom of standard ethical theories and principle for such wisdom is not in any way helpful in classifying the said problems. In fact, the act is of classification or grouping necessarily needs a *criterion or criteria*. We should better concentrate on this matter. It is difficult as I think, to classify bioethical problems on the basis of a criterion because we may need more than one standard criterion in such cases. First, it is important to base our classification on the *discovery of the imminent questions of value* (ethical) in practical problems for the health care professionals and the bioscientists, the method of which has been elaborated to some extent before. Without such "discovery" we are not able to proceed in classifying the value issues under "death and dying" for instance, as different from issues under "biomedical researches". There is a problem in this case nevertheless, as *knowing* that such and such practical problems are value-laden cannot become a basis for distinguishing one group of problems from another group unless another basis has been found for such distinction. Second, there is need to speak about *nature of the theoretical-practical* (or technical) aspects of these problems because when we take care of such things, it is not difficult to ascertain why "abortion" should be grouped under the first group of problem (death and dying) as distinct from the second one (biomedical researches). More interesting is to notice that the first and now the second basis of classification of problems are closely related as together they lay stress on the "queerness of practical problems" and the "unique structure of their thesis", which further constitutes sets of value-questions of dissimilar nature. Hence, though there is no logical deduction of "ought" from "is" involved in discovering and distinguishing value-laden issues, there is no "naturalistic fallacy" either, though there is little doubt about the synonymy of "value questions" and "practical problems". It is too odd therefore, to think that some related things are synonymous or equivalent and that one is logically deduced or derived from another. In fact, such issues are better said, "ethical-practical", that is, a whole in which the "practical and the theoretical" go along with the "ethical" or the "value" questions – they are inseparable elements or properties, as if, of the whole of the issue. Truly, therefore, we need to group bioethical issues after taking care of both the theoretical-practical intricacies and the ethical questions of unique character they raise. Next, we have to take care of *unique relations* in which some of the biomedical problems emerge. It is clear that we consider some biomedical problems to be grouped under "patient-professional relationships" rather than "distribution of health care in our societies" based on unique relation among patient, professionals and other people. In case of biomedicine, such relations are really unique, they are unavoidable. Whereas in some cases, the *locale* becomes important, for instance, in the cases of responsibilities, duties and obligations of government and non-government agencies towards those needing distribution of health care amenities. In case of many value-laden issues in health care it is, therefore, difficult to avoid the peculiar local customs, traditions, faiths, ways of life, and social, political and economic settings. In some other cases value-laden biomedical issues are classified according to the aspect of *management of information awaiting disclosure* to the sick, the family and the public. It is not unlikely that here the elements of "relation" mentioned above is important but in such cases dominating relation is shadowed by a dominating group of people, that is, by the health care professionals. Classification of bioethical problems is also possible on the basis of research and technology, that is, on the basis of *the role modern technology* plays in case of proposed good or welfare for humans at large, who involves not only living or dying or dead humans, rather animals in large numbers. Such things cover genetic testing, genetic therapy and many reproductive manipulations with human subjects.

Keeping these things in mind we may now assert that on multiple bases bioethical problems are grouped by biologists, medical professionals and ethicists needing no cooption and dependence on ethical theories. This is an extremely technical job done by the groups of interested parties through a long time. We should now have a glimpse of the sub-issues within the broad groups or classes as has been classified on the basis of more than one criterion. We find a class of value-laden problem called: "The beginning and end of human life", which includes important sub-issues: *Abortion, Euthanasia* and *Assisted Suicide* on the one hand and *In Vitro and In Utero researches, surrogate parenting and cloning* on the other hand. Further we have another class: "Biomedical Research and Technology" which includes *researches on humans and animals, eugenics and manipulations with human genes.* Next, under the classes of "Health care" and "Public Health management" respectively, we have issues like *Just distribution of health care facilities*, the *global epidemic management* and *Risk management in clinical tests and Researches with regard to HIV/AIDS* etc. we may have another class of issues as: "Relationship among the sick persons and the health care professionals", wherein we discuss issues like *health care codes, duties and responsibilities, rights and duties of sick people, the value of truth telling, informed consent and confidentiality in information etc.* Let us be cautious about our classification and the listing of sub-classes therein – they are not complete or fool-proof or even most satisfactory. However, they are good working classifications when we deal with biomedical ethics calling most urgently for finding proper ways to resolve these value-laden problems. It is interesting is to notice that we now come to realize that keeping in view the *methodology* of resolution, there is at least another major value-laden issue, that is, "what ought to be the valuable or the ethical method of resolving value-laden biomedical problem?" To my mind, this is extremely important as having a proper method of ethical resolution is not enough, the method should be ethical itself. (See vol. 1) Let us come to this issue now.

Now that we have discussed about the discovery of value-laden bioethical problems and the ways in which such problems may be grouped, we come to the problem of "resolution of value-laden or ethical issues in biology and medicine". This is however a tricky affair, most probably the most tricky aspect of bioethics because regardless of the importance of finding out ways to live a good life, it is a matter of finding out methods of living a good life by means of keeping away moral dilemmas troubling many sick people, their families, friends, acquaintances and the responsible body of health care professionals. In fact, we have been gifted with uncanny power to find out methods of resolving moral dilemmas, which itself becomes matter of scrutiny because not all methods discussed by us are logically sound and practically helpful. Some methods are utopian, not of much use and some others are too cumbersome filled with jargons. A straightforward method, which is logical, justifiable, pragmatic and useful, should be "ethical" as well because some methods are "unethical" in so far as they are heavily theory-laden and call for *group-chauvinism* or narrow demands for expertise at the cost of leaving out wider demands for *social interaction*. A loss of social interaction is unhealthy for biomedical science for it is loss of information to resolve some nagging crises.

Yet, "methods" we must have for our present purpose. The most "dominant method" of resolving morally charged issues which is debated strongly in our societies owing to wide disagreements is to depend on *expert* ethicists and/or biomedical scientists. We may say that the dominant method begs "ethical expertise" or "ethical engineering". This method naturally calls for people "expert" in theories of ethics, ethical codes and principles and to find out which theories, codes and principles suit best to which situation, that is, to which practical problems so that there are no more moral disagreements and we are able to frame some *decision-making rules* for health care professionals in particular so that they take morally responsible decisions in health care in the near future. The supporters of the "dominant model" hold that there is no logical possibility of finding out what "should" or "ought" to be done, that is, what is ethically desirable, in case of biomedical trifles unless we have serious *ethical theorizing* with regard to what "is" the case. Hence, practical affairs causing ethical dilemmas should be resolved if and only if we take recourse to "ethical theories" and "ethical theorizing". The basis of such argument is that no moral 'ought to' should be derived purely based on what is the case but based on what theories propagate about "what should be done". This is what Kieffer has to say: "Clearly, we are in need of an ethic that can clarify moral dilemmas and resolve conflicts. It should be clearly understood at the outset that a transaction from 'is' to 'ought' cannot be made without inserting a value judgment independent of the fact that 'is'. It would seem that we need to engage in ethical theorizing that is responsive to current needs. Whatever role may be – *concerned lay citizens* (my italics), medical practitioner, scientific researcher, and patient – we need *principles* (my italics) to help us in this rapidly advancing theoretical-logical society."[4] What Kieffer says is extremely interesting but I have some reservations. First, there is no *strict logical* sense of "derivation" or "deduction" from "what is" to "what ought to be" by introducing an "ethical element" in such "deduction". Why at all should we think that resolution of moral disagreement in biomedical affairs is logical deduction from "is" to "ought"? We all know the latent errors in deriving is from ought and ought from is. We also have a bad habit to be obsessed with the naturalistic fallacy in case of strict logical definition of value-terms and with the logical deduction of ought from is. We believe that in any case where practical affairs are judged for their ethical value, naturalistic fallacy has been committed. If we go by what Frankena and others have said [*cf.* Cross and Woozley (eds.), *The Republic*], when we have not at all logically defined an ethical term, there is no definist fallacy, and when there is no logical deduction in the true sense of the term, there is no fallacy of deriving ought from is. Hence, it is not necessary and sufficient to argue that bioethical issues causing moral dilemma should be resolved by an ethical theory to save us from any fallacy of deriving ought from is. We have argued at length that a biomedical problem ("is") does not become an ethical problem at the same time ("ought") by virtue of any ethical theory – the idea is absurd. Some problems (about what is) are value issues as well for different reasons. Our moral experiences in daily social intercourses help us in realizing these issues, that is, in knowing that some so-called stark practical affairs are inherently moral affairs as well – the issues are thus inseparable. Hence, we do not "logically deduce" any ethicality from what is. Further, our urge to solve these moral dilemmas to live a good life does not beg an ethical thesis because I will argue shortly that no ethical thesis can stand out as a premise in a strict logical argument when we take on applying our ethical knowledge (not ethical theories) to fulfil the said noble urge. I would try to show that resolution of moral dilemma does not require a method of strict logical argument. This becomes clearer when we find that Kieffer realizes well (and I appreciate) that resolution of bioethical dilemmas or disagreements need "concerned" people – "the lay citizen" and others who are not ever aware and trained about the logic of moral discourse to find ought from is. The whole affair of logic is extremely technical, the best way is not to demand such technical knowledge from lay-people who are nevertheless perfectly equipped with rich moral experience and knowledge and thus competent for moral resolution. In fact, moral resolution transcends strict logic in a moral discourse with the public for informal arguments and heuristic acumen help untrained people in logic to be logical about ethical matters.

It is perhaps more interesting to notice that though Kieffer recognizes the value of public discourse in resolution of bioethical issues; he speaks of a "methodology" of resolution which does not free itself from being theory-laden and expert-based. He states clearly that "Humans develop their ethics by the method of public discussion leading to public acceptance of what appears to be right and good and a rejection of that which is judged to be wrong or bad. Further, our conception of what is ethical, right and good changes in the light of new knowledge and continuing debate. Using these tactics, societies can develop effective ways of sanctioning the uses of new knowledge and technology even when these uses initially conflict with existing societal or individual legal, moral, or religious ones".[5] What Kieffer asserts here is of worth, he is truly bringing out the value of people's participation in resolution of tricky bioethical matters but what follows from his earlier assertion, the objectionable part is the use of "ethical theories". However, he further says that such resolution of ethical matters is never final because we do not perceive all alternatives and all consequences of the future. But there is no doubt that ethical decision-making needs a sound method, which is the crucial matter for our debate now.

What Kieffer, myself and others have in mind in this context is that ethical resolution and decision-making of value-laden biomedical issues involves "application of ethics" particularly applying ethics in "professional decision-making" and for that matter we have a complex situation of applying ethics, both needing a sound "methodology". The crucial matter therefore is to clearly state what applying ethics consists in when it comes to professional matters or else much confusion is in the offing; one among them is to take theory-cooption necessary to apply ethics in professional matters. Kieffer draws our attention towards the three major bioethical positions with regard to the application of theories of ethics, namely, *contextualism*, *consequentialism* and Kantian *deontology*. It is here that Kieffer is explicit in the statement of method of applying ethics for ethical decision-making in such matters in terms of applying standard normative theories by "concerned people". It is queer nevertheless how this methodology would justify the way layman knows and applies these intricate theories with many others. Anyway, let us find out an answer in the three major positions called, the *Proportionate Good School*, the *Prohibitionist School* and the *Rawlsian Contractualism*. In addition to a critical survey of these views, I would like to discuss what Beauchamp and Walters hold in a worth noticing "Introduction to Ethics" in *Contemporary issues in Bioethics* (1959).

The "proportionate good" thesis has been advocated by the author of erstwhile famous *Situation Ethics*, Professor Joseph Fletcher. He is known widely for his "contextualistic utilitarian" position in *Situation Ethics*. Professor of medicine, Mr. Fletcher holds that the evaluation of intentional human acts as "good" and "bad" are based on the favourable and the unfavourable or the beneficial and the harmful *consequences* of the actions on people and society at large. Such "consequentialism" amounts to hold view about decision-making in practical affairs, which is the "proportionate good", that is, the *principle* advocating the decision of some such actions or remedies (as in medicine) depending on the intricacies of the changing *contexts* which are proportionately maximizing good over evil for the general "well being" of the person (or patients). Hence, in medical parlance, that is positively good decision over evil and thus right and just over wrong and unjust which are contextually speaking, a positive means or conditions for the end, that is, well being of the patient. Any therapy therefore is judged to be medically and ethically good and right which produces good consequences for the patient and not bad ones. Taking this to be his basic "principle" Fletcher calls for ethical remedies to medical dilemmas of issues like abortion, In Vitro conceptions, cloning and other things though we must not forget that the end being good-itself, that is, "well-being of patients", the *means* are worth considering, for our practical decisions for "therapy" needs to be or *should* be good as well. Therapy as such cannot be so much so evil if it is never conducive to the end in consideration. But whether or not such is the case *in reality* is a matter of calculus of the consequences or the effects to be seen in case of the patient and therefore, not to be instantly known. It is clear that the idea of means *necessarily and sufficiently* justifying end may not be a true thesis as end would not be *necessarily and sufficiently* seen as justifying means or that any end will justify a therapy (the means). If the end is egoistic pleasure maximization, deciding to give costly doses of vitamins to a wealthy may be questionable though his or her proportionate increase of fat deposition may be no decrease in his or her purse. But Fletcher has to presuppose that we have a physician of good will and who is rational enough for deciding what is proportionately good for welfare of patient. Several questions crowd in our mind but we have to be more careful. For Fletcher, though well-being is the desirable end for patients, means, such as the acts of therapy, may be flexible. It would be foolish for physicians to follow a stringent absolute code of conduct imposed by an authority to not to inflict physical harm in any case. If we follow this "noble means", perhaps our good intending surgeons have to give up their job of cutting flesh. Hence, there is no place of absolutism in medical decision-making of what ought to be done now because factuality cannot be overwhelmed by sheer *a priori* conception of "this must be right". Taking this, though we aim at welfare, aborting a woman for she carries a girl child who is likely to be neglected after birth in her family, may not be a "good decision". Or, not aborting a woman who carries a deformed fetus for her well-being because deformity is not testimony to death but life may be a "bad decision". In any case, "good" and "bad" in these contexts are of ethical relevance. Fletcher comes to conclude that for a valuable ethical decision-making (or choice of means that is good) might take a cue from pragmatic guidelines of compassion, consequence, proportionate good, actual need than ideal, enlarging choice and reducing chance and responsible to make decisions. We must keep in mind ultimately that physicians' decision-making should be in view of the ethical theory of well-being or biological welfarism.

All this is very good but there are certain problems which we face. First is that in any given situation or context a physician of 'goodwill' must be aware of one ethical theory necessarily and sufficiently for that is the "end theory", the absolutely true one. We are not raising any doubt on the call of "well-being" of patients; we are just mentioning that the thesis may not be the only one thesis in evaluating medical decision-making. Fletcher has rightly recognized some degree of "relativism" in the choice of proportionately good decisions in a situation. The problem is why "well-being" is the only ethical theory needed for such evaluation? Interesting things crops up when we ask more questions: How do we come to know that our noble doctor has "goodwill" and not an evil one? Is determination of "having goodwill" helped by decision of good means or desirable end or both? Can decisional act be a testimony to "having goodwill" or we have to wait for effects and then judge for goodness? Is the entire affair not clumsily future dependent? Or, do we fall back on *a priorism* and/or intuitionism for determination of goodwill? Fletcher does not answer many of these questions properly. For me, however, the most important question is to ask Fletcher whether or not it is practically feasible or possible or even desirable for a physician or other concerned people to keep an eye on welfarism while choosing what to do now which is conducive to good over evil produced? To my mind, the whole affair is not only unpragmatic, it is unethical because fixity of mind in ethical-theory-cooption is in itself derogatory to *apply* medical persons' ethical knowledge of good and desirable undetermined by academic knowledge of ethics. Application of physicians' ethical knowledge of end of life and deciding to do good and not bad, and the welfare of other beings and things is perfectly possible when we believe that theory cooption is an exclusively technical affair needing trained ethicists and/or medical experts trained in academic ethics. Further, it is over-demanding from our imaginary computer-programmed physicians, the "moral engineers", to pick up "this theory only" for "this case now" and decide "this for good". It is not understandable why rather than "welfarism", deontological theory is not called upon service to judge production of proportionate good over evil. Or, to press "theistic ethics" to do the same. Most queer is, does physicians and health care professionals know these theories, their justifications and choose them in a mechanical way? Is it not important to care for the disagreements emerging among many people about decision-making? They may want seriously to produce good over evil for human welfare and to find out ways to move out of such stiff impasse through corroboration of views, which Kieffer does recognize? What Kieffer and Fletcher forget is that public involvement in ethical resolution is vital for value-resolutions in biomedicine without theory cooption and ethical engineering. The "unethicality" of the model mentioned here is that moral chauvinism rules supreme in value-resolution of biomedical issues. Theory cooption and obstinately clinging to medical chauvinism is not at all healthy. We cannot grossly neglect the moral opinions of women of various strata and emotive states, their associates and other people when it comes to resolution of moral problems in abortion and merely fall back on physicians and their chosen clan-thesis in the name of either public ethics or private ethics.

Does the "prohibitionist model" help us in this regard? The model finds support in the writings of Paul Ramsey who is a Christian ethicist, the author of works like *The Patient as Person* (1954) and *The Ethics of Fetal Research* (1975). In these works he proposes something different from Fletcher because he believes that for the sake of human welfare any means cannot be taken as good itself. It is due to this that in medicine several decisions may be taken, mostly experimental and therapeutic which can be done easily given our technological and other advances, but not ethically desirable. Similarly there are some such things which can be known but should not be known and applied. For instance, given present knowledge and technological advances, we can easily experiment on fetus and manipulate with genes but rather becoming great advantages or producing well-being, they are intrinsically evil or undesirable as means because they induce a number of ethical problems for mankind than solving them. Ramsey argues that experiments on fetus for instance induces moral problems of desirability of non-therapeutic abortion and trespasses moral authority of an experimenter to unconsented manipulation with fetus and cause damage to potent life (the fetus). These ethical issues cannot be and should not be solved by the guidelines given by Fletcher, that is, by weighing the proportionate good over evil for human welfare. In this place, Ramsey thinks that we should weigh the case of fetal research in totality or in its entirety, which covers the social and moral prices we have to pay for the said research. According to Fletcher a careful calculus of the touted "benefit" or "well-being" *vis-à-vis* the price we have to pay for it amounts to more of cost than benefit. Hence, for ethical decision-making a care for social and moral concerns or the cost people have to pay should overwhelm mere physical "benefits". Fletcher thinks that if production of good over evil is important to a great extent, then many of our medical decisions for choice of means needs ethical scrutiny for their rejection, such as euthanasia, genetic research and experiments on humans. Whatever may be the Kantian overtone in Ramsey, what interests us most is that for him principles of universal character and acceptance need to be emphasized for the resolution of moral impasse in modern medical decision-making. These are the principles of "sacredness of human life" and "conventional relation among physicians and sick people". These are truly imported ideas from Christian theology with some Kantian bearings such as "respect for person". Though the ideals are often adverse to what we find in practical situations, Ramsey would like to see them succeed by virtue of proactive application by the physicians' community and the ethicists.

One wonders what is new in Ramsey when the point is not of end and means rather of proving a point of application of standard ethical principles in order to resolve moral crises which he has mentioned. Let us not contest here the defects of Kantianism and Theological ethics; here we should be reasonably concerned about how Ramsey's basic principles may be applied by concerned parties. Our reply is that those principles cannot be applied in the perceived artificial fashion. I would like to find out cases when the persons in "covenant", if they are not mere dummies in relations but equally important, allow on moral grounds that at least one party applied a theory, and the other one supplies a problem and then awaits resolution. The "covenant" cannot allow a "division of labour" as the physicians and the ethicists solve problems on the one hand for they are knowledgeable experts of ethical principles and the sick people are onlookers. If dignity of life is really important, how can patients' and other persons' non-theory coopted views be not taken into consideration? Moreover, even if "life" is not "sacred" in the theological sense rather biologically valuable, and if "respect" for it is replaced by "commitment for well-being" what great harm will be done? Most trifling is, there is an artificial division of labour in application of ethics which is unacceptable. Let us drop this therefor.

When we come to John Rawls' theory, which is an amalgam of consequentialism, Kantian deontology and contractarianism in his *A Theory of Justice* (1972), the idea of a contract or covenant between moral agents has not diminished. Even the traces of deontology of Kant with some risky consequentialism (most queerly) linger as well. Despite the application of this thesis in economic affairs, particularly in resolving ethical crisis in this field, it finds a place in biomedical ethical decision-making (no less queer). Whatever the peculiarity of placing Rawls may be, what we get from the thesis is that in situation of social covenant (as in therapeutic relationship), free, rational persons ought to choose principles of "justice" from an "original position" of "equality" putting a "veil of ignorance", as if, when they do so to ignore the tensions among social, economic and political factors influencing choice, the rational agents become free to apply the theory of "justice in original position" to dispel many ethical doubts in biomedicine, particularly those about distribution of health care benefits. It is difficult to find out what Rawls' theory could do in order to resolve cases of abortion and euthanasia, if we take him in the real context but more problematic is to find out the way our poor doctors, nurses, ethicists (perhaps not one who wants abortion) be in an "original state" of "ignorance" to do "justice". It may be highly debated and found undesirable for any of the concerned parties in medical decision-making to put a veil on contextual truths, the socio-political and economic tensions to resolve the crises of non-therapeutic abortion. How can these people come to a queerly metaphorical "original state" in case of biomedical impasse is very difficult to understand. Moreover, why this principle should be applied and not any other in state of originality is impossible to understand. To block ethical pluralism along with non-experts' participation in dissolving ethical crises is a bad habit on our part.

Our line of attack on unfounded "principlism" and "artificial models of ethical application" in biomedicine is well recognized by Tom Beauchamp and Le Roy Walters in *Contemporary issues in Bioethics* (1999). They aptly put it as follows: "One possible response to the problem of public moral dilemmas and disputes is that we do not have and are not likely ever to have a single theory or method of resolving public disagreements. In any pluralistic culture there may be many sources of moral value and consequently a pluralism of moral points of view on many issues…however, there also are ways to alleviate at least some moral dilemma and disagreements".[6] This is perfectly in tune with what I want to stress in application of ethics. No doubt, ethical issues are complex; they involve many parties and not many moral theories. In fact, an artificial application of any one or more theories is extremely problematic than a great benefit. The question is: If our editors are so sure about "ways to alleviate" these problems, what they are? In a following section (p. 4 of their edited work), they initiate a lengthy discussion under "The Resolution of Moral Disagreement". They call for an agglomeration of methods making perhaps a whole or a model, which we shall try to unravel. The first 'method' is to obtain "objective information" because for lack of many current *non-moral* information from the vast progresses made in biomedicine, ethical theory and principles themselves or our urge to deliberate on moral issues does not make much progress. Undoubtedly, it is futile to conceive of a public debate on compulsory screening for HIV/AIDS without being well informed about the current information we have about this matter. The information needed is about degree of knowledge to be gathered by screening, the risks of public health and about the role of sex campaign and education. Hence, one way to spread out our method from the confines of moral engineering is "gathering relevant biomedical information". Further, we have the method of "providing definitional clarity", that is, we must be clear about what exactly we mean by "abortion" and "euthanasia" before we start dealing with its ethic. There is much complexity in this as any fixed idea about these things might lead us to a fixed set of ethical judgment or to no valid judgment at all. Next, we should "adopt a code", that is, to come to a common agreement on a set of moral guidelines so that emerging disagreements about a moral impasse can be comfortably resolved. In fact, if belligerent parties are left to stick to their moral views, perhaps there can be no moral decision-making. It is in this respect that our editors mention about the much discussed "principles of respect for persons", "beneficence" and "justice", which are important starting points in resolving biomedical crises by the commissioners bestowed upon to do the jobs. We further have the method of "using examples and counterexamples" in order to resolve bioethical issues again by the appointed people or the experts so that the history of medical cases and counter-cases may be elaborately discussed to find out whether or not, for instance, euthanasia is morally permissible, the three basic principles mentioned above notwithstanding. Finally, the method seeks "analyzing arguments" so that gappiness in different moral positions could be exposed and rejected, whereas sound ones gives way to formulate decision-making rules. This is expectedly an intricate philosophical affair. The honest editors conclude by saying that: "Our pragmatic goal should be a method that helps in circumstances of disagreement, not a method that will always eradicate problems".[7]

I agree largely with what Beauchamp and Walters hold because their methods rolled into one come out to be an excellent model for public participation in ethics. However, I find some problems in their version knowing fully well that they do not have any intention to build methods rather, what they have found is empirically based or based on their profound knowledge as ethical decision-makers. What is objectionable is that the proposed model falls short of "public participation" in ethical resolution because there are traces of undesirable "principle cooption" as well as dependence on "moral expertise". The public is really neither "three principle co-opted" necessarily and sufficiently nor are they expert "commissioners". Commissioners make public but the "public" is not merely "commissioners". Three principles are equally not the only basis for our wise "commissioners" to channel moral decision-making for they have perhaps least regard, as I believe, for the "other parties", the sick, their associates, the family and many others who are not trained in "three principles" and "commissioning" moral views. These "other parties", nevertheless, are good debaters and my experience in this field tells me that all "three" principles and many more could be seen as effective in public discourses for finding out moral agreements. Moreover, despite stiff differences in moral thesis avowedly pet to people, (even the opposed ones), really fizzles out when ethical corroboration comes to the fore. Apparently opposed ethical thesis is found astoundingly supportive of *one decision* to be taken in the final run. Perhaps theoretic differences or clinging to a thesis affects "*how* something ought to be done" but more often than not they are on the same footing about "*this* should be done". I find no reason to suppose that a staunch follower of Kantian deontology when comes closer to a utilitarian regarding the ethical role of the government agencies in distributing health care to the poorest of the poor, would at all fight for justifying that such care should be either provided or not provided. It would be nevertheless, a matter of careful study the way these theory coopted people are suggesting *ways to provide such care* to the said group and to *what extent*. Even if belligerent debaters are non-philosophers and non-scientists, they would perfectly follow two lines of thought most unknowingly and yet, come to corroborate ethical views about the broader resolution for decision than finer disagreements for technicalities involved., Perhaps the lingering problems of ethical dimension, which truly our editors mark out as obstinate, never to be finally solved, is due to this "precision element" in moral discourses.

This brings us to statement of the "model" I propose in this regard and the value of ethical theories and principles in this regard. Strangely though, our editors move on with the truth in moral relativism but comes to both standard theories and principles of ethics as well as some known anti-theoretic or anti-principlistic thesis knowing fully well that public scrutiny of moral impasse may not need principles and theories. But for this, first we should agree that public participation model is in any case not tantamount to participation of a few people or some experts. If chauvinism is in bad taste in ethical resolution, "commissioners" cannot be the sole party as doctor and ethicists are not. If we imagine that a governmental or non-governmental agency allows the covenanted commissioners to talk to the suffering people and the health care professionals of a nation, the ethically oriented talk is an "one to one" contact or "one and a small group contact", not a moral debate rather professing and collecting information. There is least doubt that if we progress along with the professed model of "mass contact" made by an expert or experts in biomedical ethics, they would collect things like "three principles" or "some theories" or "some virtues and values" but it will be difficult to determine what disagreements might emerge about these principles, theories and virtues and values when mass is not merely contacted and professed but liberated to debate on moral matters. Our greatest problem is that though application of ethics is best when it faces tough situations, we have to find out which "tough situations" call for such a good name. The point here is one of facing tough talking people among a milieu of moral principles, theories, virtues and values emerging and blowing out or, some of them are cared by these concerned parties as most important. Among people, ethics-talk is not one of selection of principles, theories, virtues and values merely; the straight point is to solve crises within theoretic turmoil. Once we do this, there is no wonder to find a Kantian, a utilitarian, a casusist and a principlist churn out some "ought", though none of these ordinary people belong to any of these esoteric coterie of ethical philosophers because moving away from expertise, chauvinism, professing, information gathering and commissioning, practical resolution of bioethical issues are best found in "real dynamics" of application of our ethical knowledge (not of theories) to solve value-laden issue. Precisely, "face divergent groups together to know how to resolve bioethical crises" may be the point; there is nothing great in theory cooption and manipulation.

The volumes of works on bioethics, each stressing on "try this to solve this" because "we found that this jigsaw fits that" may be completely out of reckoning lest least regard is for what people argue about. In fact, there has been a gross neglect to confuse two categories in bioethical resolutions, that is, the "analysis of post-debate findings" and "application of ethics through debates and talks". To be clear, it is one matter to put our whole effort on arranging ethical debates so that our ethical knowledge are pressed into service for resolving an issue and it is another matter to churn out theories, principles etc. from the debates. More dangerous however is to stop debates any further on the ground that theoretical tools for resolving problems have been found, and for that reason, we may now take them as means of convenience henceforth. What is great about the theories and principles churned out in discourses and trying some kind of expertise? What would be great in advocating, propagating and writing about numerous theories and principles and the ways they might be helped? When ethics has not been really "applied", post application wisdom is bereft of value. Application of ethics in biomedical matters is an ongoing process – it does not and need not stop somewhere. The *academic* value of theories and principles are never lost, there is no need to trash or stop them either but in any case the dynamics of applying ethics at the public level must not stop. Theories must not rule application from the top. Let us not give too much value to ideas like: "take this theory, it was very useful in solving euthanasia when we talked to people, and now apply them in any case of euthanasia without much worry". The theory and anti-theory debates would thus go on and on for eternity, the fight for lost grounds by casuistry and theological ethics will continue and many noble principles and virtues are found, but pray, we better not stop our good habit to take a case in and with the public as and when needed for resolution. The more we do this, the more we apply ethical knowledge, amounting to great learning. Application of ethics in professional turmoil is a 'learning process'.

Few years back I delivered a lecture to some select audience, mostly psychiatrists, students of psychiatry and other people about the way in which we can deal with the nagging ethic of use of placebos. I was advocating the model of "intersubjective corroboration", the corner stone of people's ethics, when a participant asked a wise false question: "Do we have to talk to concerned parties in hospitals and elsewhere when some distilled water needs to be pushed to a patient troubling much for high doses of Calmpose?" If this is application of ethics, well, god, save us. All showed some teeth without even an idea that the continuity of application of ethics does not mean that doctors, nurses and the sleepless poor guy needing calmpose, sat for a brainstorming. For instance, Kant says, "We must do our duties but let us tell the maniac the truth". Or, Mill says, "This would not maximize good over evil in human society, let us tell this to our maniac".

Dear readers, "intersubjective corroboration" advocates debates in and with the public about "placebos", for instance, *not every time* but *sometimes* to be sure because decisions filtered that way are good for the treating and caring public as well as for the patients but any amount of satisfaction that we had enough wisdom might be foolish and, therefore, some care for debates as and when any emerging disagreements are too sharp among the health caretakers and the public, is surely needed. Who knows, another round of resolution would not give us something better? The progress of biology and medicine is phenomenal, if Dolly the sheep raised ethical questions when she was cloned, we raise fresh set of ethical questions when she developed arthritis. Did we resolve them forever? Most likely not, hence, there is need for *corroborating* our moral views on raging ethical issues at important epochs of human history. I have said in *The Primer* (vol. 1) and at many places that resolution of problems like bioethical problems is a matter of knowing the ethically desirable model of resolution, that which is proactive, pro-people but not chauvinistic. It needs ethicists and physicians and other people interested in knowing and applying ethics which consists of *selection* of value-laden biomedical issues (we have talked about it), *framing* ethical questions, *arranging* moral dialogues by careful selection of concerned parties, *debating*, finding out *ways* out of dilemma, *formulating* decisions which have a human face and then going for some *academics*, that is, *post-corroboration* analysis of dialogues for finding out the *real dynamics* of theories, principles, virtues and values known and unknown to us. It may be good enough to write about the dynamics to show that ethics is not handmaid of experts and expert knowledge of a field, it is better to apply our knowledge of good, right, desirable, just, obligation, duty and so on so that best could be done than suffer in dilemma. This is possible because without knowledge of academic ethics, applying our ethical knowledge stemming from the biotic community is possible. Academic ethicists should be rest assured that they do have very important things to do for there must be at least one initiator of dialogues, analyst of views and teacher, of such application of ethics. We must be rest assured that only teaching all this may not make us great people unless we get involved in such effort. The rest of the book is all about some ethical issues in biomedicine and the way "intersubjective corroboration" works. However, persons interested in academic aspects of biomedical ethics should have some knowledge of the practical problems which await resolution and the basis of how ethically oriented questions are constructed to start dialogues. This is not 'chauvinism' or 'structuralism' because framing ethical questions is itself a matter of knowing many things from common people because it is always important to gauge the way untrained people should be put ethical questions before an organized ethical debate. Moreover, knowing biomedical theories and ethics to frame question is not 'structuralist' as it does not amount to act from the top but it is down to earth, it is proactive and pro-people. Academic ethics and biomedical ethics, along with initial rounds of "talks" with non-scientists and non-philosophers about bioethical matters are always useful in structuring a good questionnaire for an ethical debate.

NOTES

1. Kieffer, G.H., *Bioethics: A Tesetbook of Issues*, Addison Wesley, Massachusetts, 1979, p. 48.
2. *Ibid*, p. 43.
3. *Ibid*, p. 43.
4. *Ibid*, p. 44.
5. *Ibid*, p. 44.
6. Beauchamp, Tom and Le Roy Walters, (eds.), *Contemporary Issues In Bioethics*, Wadsworth, Belmont, 1999, p. 4.
7. *Ibid*, p. 6.

3

Ethical Issues in Care

It is clear by now that though biomedical ethics is closely associated to practical and professional ethics, unlike these fields it has something unique to do. Unlike practical ethics, it does not deal with a range of valuc-laden practical issues and their resolution, rather considers those issues emerging exclusively in the fields of biology and medicine for resolution, which broadly speaking, are of great concern for our health care professionals. Unlike professional ethics, biomedical ethics does not merely take up moral dilemmas troubling our professionals in various fields, rather those troubling our health care professionals. However, it takes up moral dilemmas of the sub-professionals such as nurses, medical researchers, drug specialists, drug manufacturers as well as medical attendants and the workers contributing to health care of the masses. More than this, biomedical ethics is extended up to moral dilemmas faced by common people, the subjects of experiments, surrogate mothers, animals, a fetus, a dead or a dying person and even the NGOs and governmental agencies responsible for health care decisions, allocation and distribution. Biomedical matters of such grave and broad expanse should be thus viewed as extremely important. However, the "method" of resolving the number of value-laden issues in biomedicine should be the same as applicable in other practical matters. This is what I have called "Intersubjective Corroboration" consisting of moral dialogues among concerned people of our societies followed by resolution through consensus and post-corroboration analysis of moral views.

I have provided some bases for classifying a number of value-laden biomedical issues in the earlier chapter but for all practical purpose I am not able to consider them here at one place, though I would like to take up at least four issues of great concern to demonstrate the pragmatics of applying ethical knowledge of ethicists and non-ethicists towards resolving these impasse through moral dialogue. In this chapter I would like to consider the ethical dilemmas regarding care of some ailing people who pose much risk for the health care professionals in particular and for the society at large as well as the care of the helpless such as the orphans and street people. There are some reasons to initiate the discussion by selecting the ethical dilemmas in health care. First is the value and importance of human life on earth, with whose physical and mental well being biological sciences, particularly the medical science is concerned. In the field of medicine, we cannot downplay the value of human well-being. Once we come to this aspect, our attention is naturally attracted to the number of ailing people, the physically and mentally challenged and the medically deprived masses. We all feel that such ailments leading to inevitable loss of precious life is not good, that is, it is not in anyway practically good for a nation. Though I feel some hesitation in terming "humans" as "resources", still the economical conception makes us feel the same, that is, unnecessary harm and loss of resources are not good but practically bad for a nation as a whole. The biological and the ecological values of human life are also well known to us, and we will hardly disagree on the point that ailing, suffering and losses do not contribute positively to the entire ecological community or to the biotic life. Hence, either means have to be found to prevent ailments and losses of human life or they have to be treated and cared or both should be done. This takes us to the issue of "care" and "cure" in medical ethics. Here we are not worried about the care of other animals though that is equally important, we are here concerned about the ways in which people's health care management might be more effective without any derogation of ethical face. If medical fraternity, in fact, concerned about it, we cannot skip the issue, rather consider it at the outset. One might wonder at this because to many of us more important issue should be the beginning of human life and the ethical concerns in it but a careful thought reveals that without basics of a care for human life and care for the welfare of those responsible for the human progeny, the issue of researches, genetic issues and others cannot be taken up at the outset. This is the second reason for considering the issue of care as primary. Further, it is essentially important for our bioscientists and medical persons to protect human lives from different biological threats ever lurking around and thus prolong human life span. Hence, any discussion pertaining to death, dying and killing raising ethical questions can never be more important than questions of life and living. It is due to this that one gives more importance to problems regarding health care in biomedical ethics. Next, when we come to health care profession, without glorification of the profession, we can say that the health care professionals have noble "service based ideal" as all professionals have. The "ideal" in health care profession is expectedly "wholesome care" of mankind without any disregard to other animals, living beings and the environment in which we live. Hence, the ethical problems concerning "care" should be considered as extremely important. Finally, bioscientists and medical professionals have serious social responsibilities, duties and obligations (also rights) for they are social beings, mostly "covenanted" in either an organization or an institution or at best in an association/council. The prime responsibility, duty and obligation are related to "care". It is due to this that any ethical dilemma about care of humans should be taken primarily in bioethics. I think that other thinkers might find out some other reasons for ethical concern about health care but without much fuss I would like to assert that in recent times some ethical questions regarding this matter have become prominent. Perhaps, one of the reasons for focusing on the ethical issue relating to the care of "high risk group of ailing people" (HRGs) is the rise of AIDS menace along with those of Hepatitis B and other highly contagious and life threatening diseases. Cases of cancer care may be included as well. It is strange if some of us do not understand that a covenanted professional doctor or nurse is not to sacrifice life as part of his or her duty. What is good is losing precious professionals by being foolhardy? Hence, we need to take "care" of the lives of our professionals when they take care of HRGs. The complexity of the issues grows more and more when some tough ethical questions start pouring in. We need to take care of these questions in our times. It is due to this that in this Chapter, I shall consider resolution of ethical questions pertaining to the care of the HRGs. Not only this, in modern times, the demographic complexities have challenged us to take care of the physically and mentally challenged people as well as to take care of the helpless people, the orphans and the street dwellers. We cannot avoid the problem of equitable and/or reasonable distribution of health care to such people in civil societies, which is, however, a tricky affair for our health care professionals. Given these reasons, therefore, let us start with the value-laden biomedical issue of health care to the HRGs, the physically and mentally challenged people and the helpless people in our societies.

The discussion henceforth follows a set pattern. First, we shall briefly explain the important aspects of public health care, the crucial issues involved in its management, allocation, distribution and the ethic of nursing as distinct from that of physicians and other health care takers. Second, we shall introduce the unique practical problems involved in the health care of HRGs, physically and mentally challenged people and the helpless people in India. Finally, I would like to explain an instance of intersubjective corroboration resulting to resolution of key ethical questions regarding this matter and analyze the real dynamics of normative theories in the moral dialogue. Statement of important decision-making rules suggested by concerned parties shall be stated as well. Let us first take up the aspects of public health care and ethicality therein.

Various aspects of public health care and the value-laden questions project one important aspect in public life, that is, unique "relationship" among the common people and the health care professionals. However, there is also a complex "relationship" among health care professionals, social and political bodies, the lawmakers, the economists, the drug companies, distributors and the ordinary ailing masses. Hence, questions of public health care is wide ranging, we ought to go for ethical scrutiny of such wide ranging matters in the backdrop of the said complex "relationship" because social good or well-being depends on maintaining a good relationship, a harmonious one to be metaphorical and not on disturbing or harming it. It is but natural that a civil society cannot evolve and grow continually if there are turmoil and hitches in intricate social relationship among those needing health care and those who provide it. To put it precisely, one basic aspect of health care is "just" and "equal" care for the masses on the whole. This may be true for all societies and times to come. In fact, if we visualize a "moral community" evolve and grow, justice in health care as well as just relationship among care takers and the needy is a must. It is needed that health care should be "impartial" because in it, caste, class, colour, creed, status, talent, abilities and fortune does not matter at all. A care for all these things over and above basic care for health gets more and more "partisan" and hinders the growth of a moral community. There would be protests, strife, violence in mind and action but not justice and harmony leading the society to divide from within. Health care, therefore, demands "impartiality"; there is no way but to serve humanity with justice. Perhaps we are in a 'social contract' – a covenant wherein stakeholders are not to be viewed in partisan ways. However, this does not rule out the possibility of "emergent" health care over "non-emergent" one or allocation of more resources in one case than in the other case. However, justice, impartiality and good relation reminds us of staying above extrinsic and intrinsic influences or pressures when cases are "emergent" and when weighing of allocations are needed. How this noble end can be achieved, which is a moral end, is the toughest question because we are continuously worried since a long time to find out ways of a non-partisan health care system. Perhaps we have not come out with flying colours, most of the time we have been defeated but we have not failed, we must try for the great ideal. May be due to this urge, we still think about "just health care". In fact, in modern civil societies, we are extremely conscious about our rights or right claims (in the sense of "due"), which enable us to envision a state of enjoying our right claims to non-partisan health care, which is qualitatively good. Hence, it is not merely for having a moral community that just health care is needed, it is "due to our good" that is needed, provided we are free citizens of a non-barbaric state governed by just laws of the land and not by subjective whim. It is good, therefore, to "claim" what is due to us if there are lack of care or, if there are exploitations by agencies. Some party, therefore, is "obliged" in health care system to respect these rights and protect them. This is needed in health care – a sense of duty towards stakeholders and obligation to a social covenant in the name of just law of the land. If in some cases the parties in the covenant feel that the legal system or a part of it is unjust itself, it needs protest, consensus and definite changes. This may not be left to the health care takers alone for the public is one party to the emergence of just laws in health care. I shall come to this aspect at a later stage. Another important aspect of health care should be highlighted here before we move on to more details about this matter. The problem in health care rights and justice is whether or not health care is as important or basic as providing "bare minimum necessities" like food, shelter and cloth. Obviously, as I have remarked before, health care does not start with mango seeds to some and mango pulp to others and then provide vitamins and irons to seed eaters and to pulp eaters in equal proportions or compulsorily to the first party. There is no doubt that health care remains a necessity, though "minimum" along with our right to good hygienic food, water, shelter and cloth. It need not be confused with providing medicines and equipments or things like that. The problem we now face more and more in status of dwindling resources and damaged environment, are really of quality living with the basic amenities and the problem of medicines, health care units, hospitals, equipments all come together when they are deemed to be necessary with good food, shelter and cloth. It is a bad habit to go for the drugs first and then mango pulp, pure water, sanitation and shelter. Yet, there are problems in the concept of what we call "decent" minimum of health care and our right claim to such thing. Allen E. Buchnan puts it nicely: "A consensus that there is (at least) a right to a decent minimum of health care pervades recent policy debates and much of the philosophical literature on health care. Disagreement centres on two issues. Is there a more extensive right than the right to a decent minimum health care? What is included in the decent minimum to which there is a right?"[1] There is some necessity to find out solution to these questions of health care, which is however, theory dependent, thinks Buchnan because without presupposing a theory of just distribution, we are unable to answer the questions of having a right to decent minimum and what are such rights. However, the theories conflict among themselves about appropriateness and logical consistency. In any case, analyzing the meaning of "decent minimum" won't help us much. Nevertheless, we should remember that our concern is not to assure basic minimum health because that is too vague to explain rather, we are here concerned about appropriate care for human health notwithstanding some broader rights for living a quality life. It must be noticed here that "having health care rights" is far different from "having and championing health care for all" or "universal health care as moral necessity" as much valuable as a matter of legal right. It would be more interesting in my mind if we enquire about "having and championing health care right" as a matter of claim right which is also morally based because a claim right need not necessarily be devoid of moral ought or else, why claim-rights as these are "desirable" or "morally good" is not known to us. Even if we do not care much for an illusory care universally or for "all", we cannot avoid the question of the moral basis of "having one claim right" because "claim rights" are not "beyond moral scrutiny". Noticeably Buchnan and others do not prefer speaking about "decent minimum health care" rather prefer to speak about "right to health care" because the inherent vagueness in "decent minimum" health care is too confusing. However, proponent of "decent minimum" thinks that any talk about "right to health care" does not take care of the relative situations prevalent in modern societies, the social, the political and the economic as well as other conditions. Hence, "decent minimum" sidesteps the more sweeping "right to health care". The notion also sidesteps the strange nature of "equal accessibility" inherent in "right to health care" and also the lack of concern for "adequately limited" care. Buchnan argues that despite these attractions, "decent minimum" is itself vague unless we presume that there is at least one fixed basis or theory to clarify what is "decent" and also "minimum" in changing social contexts, which basis may be nevertheless unfounded. Further, there is problem in finding coercive ways in distribution and governance when tendency to "decent minimum" is in principle not there but has to be brought into existence. We may reasonably accept that Buchnan speaks of a relatively conditional health care claim right in "right to health care". Hence, in biomedical ethics, when we speak of the issue of "health care" or "public health care" and the allied moral questions, we largely keep in mind this qualified sense of "right to health care" which is neither universal nor decent minimum. We need not confuse such "right to health care" with 'right to basic minimum things' for our subsistence and for our good health. Public health care issues are different from the questions of sustenance and good health but equally true is that without our existence as recognizably dignified Homo sapiens, there is no issue of "public health care".

Nevertheless, there are views in this regard which stress on the hypocrisy of "rights to health care" without recognizing the need for several "interests" and "needs" in this regard. People like H.T. Engelhardt, Jr. think that there is hardly any visible "right to health care", which is a morally based secular right to health care because it is an immorality on the part of individuals or groups of individuals or a secular authority to find coercive means to a vague ideological public health care right without any regard for what some individuals need and their affordability to satisfy their needs and interests. The talk of equal optional care which is best possible is thus averse to freedom of choice, and for that matter, diversity in public health care system regarding who should get what and how much should be taken seriously. Hence, a general right to health care need not be necessarily and sufficiently based on a social contract or covenant or coercive strictures of some social and political authorities. Engelhardt, therefore, holds that: "They (rights to health care) may therefore conflict with the decisions of individuals who may not wish to participate in and may indeed be morally opposed to realizing a particular system of health care. Individuals always have the secular moral authority to use their *own resources* (my italics) in ways that collide with fashionable understandings of justice or the prevailing consensus regarding fairness".[2] We are well aware of such health care position in the age of modernization, globalization and free market economy. Even in India, we are feeling the heat of noble "individual freedom" of choice in the large context of a huge medical market or health care business. Moreover, there are calls for "independence" in using our own resources and our entitlement to purchase best possible health care because it is another commodity to be grabbed. We have suddenly discovered that our health care marketability potential is excellent and in relation to UK, USA and other places, it is "cheap". Interesting enough is to notice that this relative "cheap" is good for people of UK and USA but not Indians necessarily. It would be an important data to find out the percentage of Indians who are "entitled" to so-called "quality health care at good price" and free to "spend" accordingly, which thus enable us to conceive a "class". Is it ethically good for us to follow the capitalist line of health care justice where care is for a class and not mass? Several intriguing questions emerge here. Extremely important is to discuss at length the ethical basis of allowing a mixed basket of health care in countries like India where mass get what they should get at the price they pay or the subsidies that do not ruin the government exchequer as well as where a class gets what they should get at the price they pay or the fund they help raise indirectly to pay subsidies. We cannot whisk one alternative without systematically and logically scrutinizing the other. This makes the value questions in health care extremely interesting. It is due to this that value questions in health care transverse the realms of political and economic decision-making in a nation. It enters the areas of debate about the ethic of the differences in entitlements of the rich and the poor, and the ethic of slowly but surely throttling the government health care bodies for flourishing of paid clinics and private health care business houses. It does call our attention to face the ethic of health care to the economically unfortunate people in terms of basic minimum but not "quality" – the problem is one of unfairness *vis-à-vis* fairness. The ethic of public health care is thus fraught with stiff questions of *models* of such care, which, I fear, though envisioned to be just and fair, is still not in view. Understandably champions of capitalist system of public health care should speak of a "multilayer" health care system (as does Engelhardt), which I believe makes a good case of public debate how the "layers" should get what they are entitled to get.

We now come to an extremely important aspect of public health care, called the aspect of "relationship" among the physicians, non-physician and patient or ailing people. Here 'non-physicians' are those care providers to the ailing people who make a heterogeneous group consisting of trained nurses, midwifes, ward boys and technical assistants. It is undeniable that when it comes to ground level public care, patients are in contact with and dependent on these non-physician care providers though their contact with and dependence on the physicians may be more primary or basic. Several ethical questions come up when patients are in "relation" with these groups for their welfare. In case of patients' well-being, it is equally important to look into the relationship among the non-physicians and the physicians, and there are interesting questions of morality to address to when we take this aspect seriously. All this is so important because we have since long cherished an *ideal relationship* among stakeholders or patients and the health care providers, who are perhaps the stockholders. Much has been written on this aspect, the ideal of great sympathizers or empathizers or even selfless and self abnegating care takers on the one hand and the ailing people, who are great admirers, placing these people only next to God and who strive with exemplary self belief to help care and cure in steady and fast manner. However, it is important to mention that the conception of an ideal patient-health caretaker relationship has not remained the same through the ages. At one time we thought our dear doctors to be our Gods, at times our saviours, still at other times our friends in need, and sometimes we related ourselves as customers, the stakeholders. It is not difficult to find out a sea change in our perception of this "relation". To many people, the relationship is or should be *feminine*, much like mother and children depending heavily on her for care and cure, and to some other people the relationship is or should be *paternalistic*, much like Freud's father who cared but stood at a distance, not participating, sharing and empathizing. We may say that patient-physician relationship is either idealized as *caring and sharing* or as *caring at a distance*. At the corporate jungle and the concrete culture, says many, the relation has been reduced to another giver and taker, one who purchases care and cure from the other at competitive cost. Here, the patient bargains, so does the doctors and nurses, and each make merry if everything is alright or, one party goes to the legal aid to sue the other. In any case, modernity and legality, the sense of rights but no obligation and duties, the pride and prejudice of wealth but not compassion has completely defaced the ideal relationship as perhaps neither maternal nor paternal but mechanical. Does morality creep in somewhere? Many say, 'yes', many say, 'no' but we have to think more. We have to think what traits of character make us any nobler that villainous and participatory than mechanical. We ask: What is desirable? What is good? What is just? In any case, if speaking about an ideal relationship among caretakers and receivers makes any sense we are bound to justify the end or the goal of public health care because without clear conception of what should be the ultimate end of health care, we cannot say that such and such relationship is desirable or just. We should be careful about the truth that patient-physician relationship is neither accidental nor fortuitous; it is a definite one lest we realize that such relationship is "goal bound" or "end directed". Hence, more than traits of character or individual virtues, like loving, compassionate, beneficent etc. it is important to look into the goal of health care keeping which in mind, a relationship grows and is said to be an "ideal" one. However, there are views harping more on inherent character traits or virtues than ends because a lack of empathy would not the least enable a physician to achieve the end of well-being of ailing people. Hence, even if well-being of patients is the cherished goal, the realization of which brings a relationship into force, lack of some human virtues in patients and physicians does not enable us to achieve the desirable goal. Many writers of managed health care thus visualize some basic elements in a caretaker-cared relationship when public physical well-being is the cherished goal to be achieved. One instance enables us to find out whether or not we agree with these elements in partiality or in totality. Hopefully, we may have some disagreement but let us have a look at the list provided by Ezekiel J. Emanuel and Nancy Neveloff Dubler: "We suggest that the fundamental elements of the ideal physician-patient relationship that are embodied in our intuitions and common to ethical analysis and legal standards can be expressed as six C's: choice, competence, communication, compassion, continuity and no conflict of interest. While many people emphasize the importance of trust in the physician-patient relationship, we believe trust is the culmination of realizing the six C's being not an independent element".[3] We may go on, as I have said, debating about these elements because some may not be in "our" intuition and some may not be in "their" intuitions. The point that is however more worth noting is the possibility of incorporating the element of "ethical scrutiny of what practical decisions ought to be taken" because all C's mentioned above are not of much worth if our population (doctors inclusive) do not take care of the resolution of moral crises in a complex relationship among the above mentioned parties. If managed care is highly methodical and not haphazard, it should find out how relations give way to moral resolutions as well. This may be treated as one essential component of managed health care which enables not only morally justifiable quality care but helps reforms within managed care. A managed health care system should be thus pragmatic, morally based and flexible to reforms through participation of concerned parties in complex "relations". However, there might be some fear perception among physician, decision-makers and others that health care reforms hinder or disparage patient-physician relationship and do not enhance it. We might thus consider this aspect in public health care. We may ask whether or not more "dedication" on the part of physicians is ethical over and above flexibility in reforms? For this however, we have to discuss the nature and method of internal reforms as I have hinted before. A reform with an ethical face need not be a threat to health care system. There is no lack of dedication in reforms if it has a human face. We shall come to these things at a proper place. In fact, archaic virtues and values may be no less damaging in managed health care if we forget that the ailing people and other people have serious social obligations, duties and honesty and dedication to display when it comes to public health care management. Why should we always tag some archaic virtues and values necessary to physicians and other health caretakers is not well known to us.

Something has been written regarding issues in public health care and the moral tensions lurking in that field. We have been particularly focusing on physicians as caretakers but we have to consider some unique issues emerging in health care when we consider "nursing" as one important aspect in health care. I have said in *The Primer* (vol. 1) that nursing should be taken as a "sub-profession" within the broad field of "health care profession" because it contributes to the professional ideal of the physicians as allies, which is the physical and mental well-being of the ailing people. However, the "sub-profession" of nursing is itself extremely valuable in attaining the said ideal. The ground reality of managed care is that major management of the sick people is at the mercy of nurses, both female and male. Consequently, there are a number of situations in ground reality care when nursing methods, means and allied technical matters are under ethical scanner. We cannot and should not skip these issues once we start discussing ethic of public health care. Issues that are most important in nursing relate to patient-professional relationship in particular in which confidentiality, truth-telling (the harsh ones) and informed consent are important. Other issues relate to cases of death and dying, particularly when nurses are faced with euthanasia, abortion and shock therapy. There is no doubt that the physicians generally face these issues in health care as the nurses but as I have said when the matter of practical application of decisions taken comes to the fore, the nurses expectedly face the brunt of moral crises and great physical and mental tension when they face the physicians, the patients, the associates of patients and the common people of society.

The unique features of nursing and ethical matters pertaining to it therefore urge for a separate treatment therefor. Many people argue that this sub-professional ethics needs a separate treatment from medical ethics though some issues as mentioned above are common to the medicos or the physicians in medical ethics. We cannot overlook two important value-laden issues in nursing ethics; these are the cases of carrying on medically necessitating orders and whistle-blowing. More often than not the orders are prescriptive in nature, in the form of imperatives that bind them to a covenanted duty and obligation, which raise moral questions of desirability or ought or should. Nurses constantly search for a resolution to their moral dilemma about necessarily carrying out these orders or to disobey them on certain ethical grounds. For instance, when a doctor orders to withdraw the life supporting system temporarily for some shortage of equipments or pressure to use it for other patients to which the attending parties and nurses do not agree on pragmatic grounds of the needs and stability of the patient in such cases, the nurse is not merely in a practical dilemma rather in a value-laden one for she searches answer to desirability, right and just. Very closely related to it is the case of "whistle-blowing", that is, a situation in which the treating physician has knowingly committed a blunder like removing life sustaining system from a not so affluent or not so important person to put it on service to an affluent or important person may be owing to some shortage of the system or for pressure, which causes death to the said patient. Or, take the case of a nurse having full knowledge of negligence of duty on the part of a treating doctor in the ICU causing unnecessary loss of life. Or, the caucus exposed for removal of kidney on operating table when the person has been attended for some other reason. The moral dilemma for the nurse is whether or not it is her duty and it is just to inform competent people or the public about the mischief? The question is when a nurse has joined her service knowing fully well and agreeing to the professional codes, rules, regulations and conditions of professional secrecy, is it ethically desirable for him or her to disclose internal bungling to the public? Equally true is that the nurses have independent codes of conduct not under the broader physicians or medical code, and for that reason, obeying orders and being forced to malpractices is not an imperative for them though keeping the greater ideal of well-being of ailing people in mind, we cannot disagree that having independent nursing code of conduct does not entitle nurses to disobey medical orders at whim or go by subjective judgments always. Whistle-blowing may be equally an offence on the part of the nurses if that becomes a potent weapon against a rightful doctor to trap him. Nursing ethics have unique features but that at best makes their sub-profession as different from medical profession but all so-called unique features and value-laden aspects are within the realm of broader managed health care that aims at well-being of people by not stressing professional hierarchies rather, essential camaraderie. Nurses are truly negotiators between medicine and nursing with some care for values. Interesting thing to notice here is that in principle, there is no way to prevent our physicians to be whistle-blowers against physicians or nurses or an evil coterie. When hierarchy becomes primary in management of health care, a physician is in dilemma to "disobey" the orders of another physician or has to "overrule" nurses' decisions, but with some ethical care.

We have just seen that codes of conduct in nursing or the nursing ethical codes are not the same as or are not under medical codes for the physicians. The question is whether or not this can be the basis of treating nursing ethics as distinct from medical ethics? Many people not supporting the distinction between the two argues that the *four principles* of *autonomy*, *beneficence*, *non-maleficence* and *justice* as suggested by Beauchamp and Childress (cf. *Principles of Biomedical Ethics*, 1989) are applicable in case of physician and nurses to resolve ethical dilemmas such as confidentiality or whistle-blowing. However, others who support essential difference between the two argue that as nursing ethics is in reality ethics of care as distinct from ethics of cure of medicine, the "four principles" might be applicable in the latter case, the former transcends them to adhere to other set of principles. Another argument in favour of distinction is that nursing ethics is in essence "feminine" as distinct from medical ethics which is essentially "patriarchic". Many feminist thinkers of our times argue in this way as does Carol Gilligan in her work *In a Different Voice* (1982). On face value the points of distinction appear to be good enough but there is enough matter for debate. The first argument is based on the idea that doctors 'cure' but not 'care', as if the first is to bodily well-being, the other, holistic, covering body and mind – the ailing person on the whole. The first is suggestive, prescriptive and imperative without a human touch, whereas the other is to the heart, tries to catch feelings and emotions with a motherly touch. It would be a good point to find out whether 'care' and 'cure' needs to be treated on these lines if public health care ought to be holistic – care and cure – prescriptive and empathetic. The other argument based on the idea of broader consideration of patient-health caretaker relationship calls for involvement of the nurses with the ailing persons, their families and associates for holistic care and cure. The relationship further extends to the caring staff and the society at large and thus transcends codes and theories. However, we may raise some more interesting questions in this context of distinguishing care, cure and feminine touch. Is it not desirable (ethically at least) to enforce the ethic of care and the ethic of feminism so to say in entire health care system including medicine and not only in nursing if all these things are so great? It may be that influenced by such an idea which is yet another misconception about care and cure, Wenz and Fletcher have advocated ethic of care and cure in medicine (*Bioethics*, 5: 3, 1991). Further, we may ask, why the principle of consideration of patients' interests be not as empathetic as the ethic of care? In any case, in health care ethics, these views and questions are of great worth.

There are some other attempts to justify that nursing ethics is distinct from medical ethics. In recent times Geralal Winslow, Mary Kohnke, Sally Gadow and others have argued that based on the idea of "advocacy" we can justify the distinction of uniqueness of nursing ethics for a separate treatment. Winslow in his paper in *Hastings Centre Report* (14: 3, 1984) holds that taking a cue from the "legal" import of "advocacy"; we need to view the efforts of the nurses as "pleaders of the case of or the good of the patients". This is to clear out of any need of principles, codes and theories about care and cure, which hopefully fall on our medical fraternity mostly. Giving another turn to this concept Mary Kohnke in her paper in *American Journal of Nursing* (80, 1980) holds that "advocacy" need not be taken as a "legal notion" rather a humanist one in which most unlike the legal advocates, the nurses act to inform and support ailing person so that he or she is able to take best decisions for revival. Sally Gadow in *Nursing Law & Ethics* (1: 8, 1980) preaches "existential advocacy" suggesting active assistance to individuals so far as their autonomy for health matters is assured. All these things are essentially different from what is expected of the physicians, resulting into a separate treatment of nursing ethics. Again there are a number of questions asking for validity of the concept of "advocacy" and subsequent independence of nursing ethics. We may ask: why in ethic of care, legal obsessions like advocacy should creep in when it does not contribute in justifying why pleading a patient's case should be taken as moral? In fact, "pleading" the case may be itself morally questionable for it does neither clarify the ethical mandate of the patient nor does it clarify the ethical role of the health caretaker in health care system. In its place, the nurse assumes the role of care at a distance by being more paternalistic as a physician. The inherent sense of "dependence" of patients on an assuming nurse for well-being may not be ethical. The imagined "autonomy" of the patient is thus defeated, as is the defeat handed over to the ideal of nursing who are not at all expected to achieve any goal through verbal or legal conflicts in managed health care. Why nurses should be taken as very enraged verbal lawyers is not known to us. Still the model raises the question of accountability to push the case of ailing people when they face neglect and mischief from any corner of the medical fraternity. In the age of consumerism we do speak of consumers well being at some cost, is it not ethically just to fix new set of responsibilities to nurses? Yet, there are fresh set of problems in so far as nurses themselves are under the legal scrutiny for any neglect and mischief because they cannot be the only "pleaders" of patients' well-being. Why should we not include physicians as well as the common public in this regard? The questions are stiff and interesting but I think there are better ways to solve them – pure theorizing may not be the best way. It is interesting to quote Ruth F. Chadwick here: "The nursing role, however, ultimately always has to be seen in a social context, because the picture of a nurse is constantly changing.

Negotiations over the boundaries of nursing are ongoing. This is why it is a mistake to try to distinguish nursing ethics in terms of one sort of problem, viz., obedience to doctors, but it is nevertheless the case that the suggestion… points to the way to what is important, namely that Nursing Ethics is essentially political. It is concerned with the dilemmas nurses have to face, it is concerned with how nurses relate to patients, but all this has to be examined within the political context of the network of professional relationship in care system and the status of nurses and women in society".[4] Ethics of care where we now stand has thus become a tricky affair. It is trickier if we now ask more stiff questions, which though avoidable, should not be avoided. We now ask: Is "care" a sufficient conception in managed health care when nursing amounts to "caring"?

In fact, such questions arise from a gamut of literature available to us on nursing and nursing ethics in which a moot issue is to find out the traditional ways of clarifying the notion of "care" *vis-à-vis* some contemporary attempts to find out what should be done rather than traditional 'caring'. Traditionally, 'caring' has been taken as a "sentiment" covering the sense of compassion, sympathy and empathy. It is also a "feeling" where a dedication to another person's well-being is needed. 'Caring' in this sense also amounts to "interpersonal intimacy" and "mutual self actualization". "Caring" in nursing is thus understood as forming a bond or a union that transcends the physical. Traditionally, to some people such 'caring' amounts to an "interactive process", an interaction among nurses and the patients through understanding, trusting, sharing experiences, ideas and knowledge. Yet, to some people professional care-taking by nurses are "cognitive ways to know the needs of ailing people and to find out scientific ways to help them".

In recent times thinkers like Milton Mayeroff and Martin Zubber have shifted from the traditional relationship among nurses and patients to find out what is more appropriate of professional nursing care. For Mayeroff, nurses' professional ethics of care is a realization of the "inner realms" of the one who needs care. Martin Bubber's conception of relationships of "I-It" and "I-Thou" helps us know that when professional health care has been taken to the level of a trans-physical, mysterious and transcendental realm of "self-realization", one experiences identity than difference. A complete abnegation of the "I" who is better placed as "caretaker" and the "It", who depends on me for "care" is in view. However, Stan Van Hooft questions whether or not such transcendentalism or mysticism is any way appropriate to a conception of professional health care because what has been said is much closer to an intimacy in "lovers' relationship" than nursing relationships. Nel Nodding in her *Caring – A feminine approach to ethic and moral education* (1984) argues that Mayeroff and Bubber must be right if "care" amounts to an engrossment, abnegation of self and becoming one with the experiences of others. However, Nodding is aware that for this health care takers such as nurses need a prolonged, constant personal relationship, which is difficult but not absurd. There are criticisms of such lofty ideal of "total encounter care" on the grounds that more often than not the care takers would find themselves as utter failures not able to penetrate upper crusts of inner spaces of patients' life and thus the ideal is unattainable. It has been asked by Helga Kushe in her article "A Nursing Ethics of Care: Why caring is not enough?"[5] Why ailing people should abide by a nursing home or hospital rules to allow nurses and other health caretakers make inroads into inner space of their life when they go there for treatment? If people do not allow such things and ask for systematic, scientific, modern and professionally competent heath care for which they pay, what unethical is done to the nursing ideal of care? Perhaps nothing at all. A professionally competent nursing often transcends catering to the physical needs when a holistic approach has been scientifically organized but for this no "engrossment" is needed. We must understand that the patients treated as "objects" of experimenting I–Thou relationship may be beyond ethical demands of privacy and individuality. It may be nevertheless desirable that nurses and patients are "open" while they make whatever fleeting relationship in a health care unit but the openness does not amount to be engrossed like love-birds.

The result of such criticism thus calls for moving beyond the hackneyed moral dispositions, moral traits, moral virtues and motivations in health care ethics because now more than "care" in this sense we deem it practically and morally necessary to become pragmatic at the theory and technical aspects of ground level caring, demanding more than affection and emotion, becomes motivated towards our professional ideal of biological well-being and thus take care of what ailing people think and do for their well-being. Most importantly perhaps, the ethic of care needs the broadening of the scope of intersubjective moral discussion about what should and what should not be done when some value-laden practical problems of caring comes to the fore. Here, in the context of moral discourse among health caretakers, particularly the nurses, the question of ethical theories and universalizable principles being applied still makes a point of debate. Many like Kushe would like to see some role of the universal ethical principles. We shall scrutinize this possibility soon but with a remark that though an ethic of health care might open opportunities for moral discourses than the fixed set of virtues and values, what fixed set of principles would do here is equally doubtful. Interestingly, one might wonder why patients with acute pain for cancerous growths should participate in any dialogue when some problem arises for the nurses to give him or her some high doses of pain-killers! Perhaps, here we do not understand the sense of "moral dialogue", which is crucial in our understanding of "care" *de novo*.

At the end of this discourse on medical health care, nursing and ethical inquiries about medical health care and nursing, we come to the problem to be considered in this work, which is the ethical problem of "caring high risk group of people, the physically and mentally challenged and the helpless people". As I have said before, these issues need a brief introduction which are said to be value-laden. I have also remarked that the ethical questions of care of the HRGs become extremely important in the context of the threat of AIDS, sexually transmitted diseases, Hepatitis etc. I would like to concentrate more on AIDS and sexual maladies in this introduction part because in our times they pose biggest challenge for management of public health. The near epidemic situation spreading like wild fire across the globe has given rise to one serious value-laden practical problem, that is, "care, cure and holistic well-being" of these "high risk group people". The physicians, nurses, pathologists and other technical and non-technical staff who are directly involved in the risky job of care and cure of these people are themselves at the receiving end of an imposing threat for their well-being and for their existence as such. No less risky is the care and cure of cancer and hepatitis B cases. Erstwhile a risky affair of care and cure of tuberculosis, typhoid, malaria, cholera, leprosy and some cases of cancer has been faced with success owing to pioneering medicine and techniques of care. Hence, as we stand now globally, the epidemic of AIDS is the real challenge for the caretakers who are presumed to be doing their duties fearlessly (but not foolishly). In fact, any talk of need of selfless, fearless and risk-taking physicians and nurses in the face of AIDS is good enough as gossips but there is no glory in our precious manpower giving away their lives without supportive research for protecting their lives from the danger they are in. Once we start thinking about such things, the welfare of care takers *vis-à-vis* receivers, many interesting value-laden questions start pouring in. I would like to give a glimpse of the value-laden practical problems here without being least technical about HIV/AIDS because such literature provided by me cannot make us any wiser. It may be nevertheless sketchily useful for some of our readers but not for the medical fraternity.

HIV / AIDS as a threat to global public health is an old phenomena by this time. We have seen nearly 25 years of this threat as it started around 1980 to spread worldwide within 12 years. Reportedly, 13 million people were infected globally with the 'HIV viruses' that cause AIDS. Later in 1997, after an estimate on HIV/AIDS, the WHO declared that 30.6 million people live with HIV infection globally, out of which 21 million live in Saharan Africa. HIV infection penetrated South East Asia as late as 1985 through Thailand. In 1992 report of the WHO, India and Thailand have maximum number of HIV/AIDS cases. By 2000, India has crossed the 5 million infected people mark and most likely to remain the worst sufferer and most potent country to spread the epidemic for its huge population in Asia and possibly a major player in the whole world. It is interesting to notice a recent local newspaper report published from Ranchi, the state capital of Jharkhand, a peaceful tribal state and still remaining relatively green by comparison with indigenous people in large numbers that nearly 35 cases of HIV infected people live within 40 kms of Ranchi, particularly around the villages of Khunti. However, the worst infected areas are expected to be near the seas and ports like Bombay and Calcutta but strangely hilly regions are no fewer sufferers owing to the drug menace. Entire north eastern states are suffering with this problem including the national capital of Delhi with a complex and shifting demographic status. The spread of AIDS is not strange as the disease is predominantly "sexually transmitted" but most unlike other such diseases like syphilis and gonorrhea, which are bacterial, and thus curable, remains incurable and uncontrollable. The disease has to spread as it is directly linked to the unstoppable human urge to satisfy sex drives and modern catastrophe of mind. Greatest problem with HIV infected people is that they live for a long course, gradually weakening infected person's immune system until secondary flare-up condition emerges, which is extremely dangerous for the caretakers and society at large. We must remember that the virus might spread in non-sexual modes as well, such as using HIV infected blood for treatment or through infected syringes, transfusion sets and through the pregnant women to the fetus they are carrying. Study in India and elsewhere reveals that rather than abusing homosexuality and drug abuse, we should point out the greatest cause of all, that is, "high risk behaviour". I must add, when we look at the public health management, "high risk caretakers" might be potent cases receiving infection in the near future. It is no more laughing a story to remember that at one time leprosy caretakers did contact the disease as did the caretakers of tuberculosis. The problem is, so far as we have no sound inoculation methods (Hepatitis B now has one), as well as drugs for care and prevention, and that we cannot throw infected people, how do we take care of such people with minimization of risk?

Writers contributing to this aspect of AIDS menace like Le Roy Walters, T.L. Beauchamp, Ronald Byre, Ferdinand Schoeman, James Childress, Minkoff, Sidney Wolfe and many others have raised important ethical issues. A glimpse of these might be useful when we further analyze the ethical discussion with some of our physicians and health caretakers regarding the problem in consideration. Many of these writers believe that ethical questions are raised mainly about policies and principles in public health care, particularly the health care of those prone to high risk behaviour, biomedical tests and researches involving such people, duties and obligations of the public and the public health caretakers, the ethical aspects of sex life, consent to care and caring the dying AIDS patients. If we go through these ethical inquiries, most of them are pertinent enough to cover the cases of care of several other risk-groups and even the disabled and the helpless but let us now concentrate on questions relating to AIDS. In so far as questions of public health care matter most, we ask whether or not it should be *ethically* "mandatory" or "voluntary" to adopt a public policy of participating in *education* of high risk behaviours as well as *checks or preventions* on such behaviours. It takes us to checks on prostitution, non-use of condoms in alien sex relations and drug abuse. It will be equally important to ask whether or not it is ethically desirable to participate in mass *screening* of blood, semen and tissues or organs as required by law. Further, it is equally important to ask whether or not public health care policies should primarily *safeguard* the welfare of the health of the health caretakers despite their social and legally necessitating duties and obligation towards all classes of people needing treatment as basic rights. It is also ethically searching though with some rigoristic fervour to ask if HIV detected cases should be provided costly health care or be systematically isolated for their misdeeds (if that be ensured). This is close to the ethic of *discriminating* one group for high risk care from another group, the discrimination for falling voluntarily in high risk behaviour than not falling into it. It is the ethic of *segregation* which is at stake here. There are questions about biomedical tests as usual, asking whether or not it is ethical to involve infected patients to laboratory tests, all sorts of mandatory tests at the cost of their self-esteem and individual freedom? Can respect be justifiably shown to sexual offenders? Serious ethical questions are about the cost-benefit analysis in AIDS research and treatment. Should countries like India and others provide costly AIDS researches and drugs to the suffering lot knowing well that the cost is covered by most people who themselves do not belong to sex and drug offender group. Interestingly, when AIDS is reaching from cities to villages, where poverty is more acute and people marginalized, should we allow expensive methods of AIDS control or subsidize it greatly or leave it to private players?

Moral questions regarding these issues are about the duty of the general public and those of the infected people as well as health care professionals. There is no doubt that if the most questioned people in health care maladies like AIDS are voluntary sexual risk behaviour people, we need to ask them about their social obligations and duties first than our questioning health care professionals for their obligations and duties. We need to ask infected people whether or not it was ethically desirable on their part to have disclosed HIV/AIDS infection, the degree and duration of infection and the sources? If infected people belong to free-sex-group or sex-workers or happen to be in trap of a sexually contacted person, is it naturally expected of them to not to go for any social contact any further even if it amounts to risk to their livelihood? Or, is it a matter of existence which should pave way to some risk-taking? Problem is also about the desirability of voluntary choice of sex partners who are confirmed cases of AIDS infection. It is a matter of great debate in "sexual ethics" that sexual life is essentially private and nothing could be as puritanical, sacrosanct and ascetically good to impose an ethic of "no sex" in contemporary world. If this be the case, why should "checks" on certain sex behaviours be desirable? Why should sex-workers' act be unethical? Why should choosing an infected partner be unethical? And why should we not allow marriage of infected partners if they so wish? More stiff questions are for health caretakers when it all falls on them to care for people who want no "checks" in sex and even marriages of infected people amounting to another infected birth causing hazard for the caretaking unit. Duties and obligations apart, should "checks" (social and legal) not precede care?

A number of ethical problems emerge in the context of testing and screening programmes of high risk group of people. The problems, as has been already hinted, lie in the mandatory *versus* the voluntary nature of tests and screening. However, many allied questions make it tougher. We may question the ethical desirability of *compulsory test* for AIDS in our societies when the infection is not transmitted through air, water and touch, thus sparing ordinary people who are careful about unsafe sex. Is it not ethically more desirable to identify those groups of people in our societies for mandatory AIDS test who are careless in sex behaviour? However, the need for compulsory test becomes crucial when it has been found that certain methods of screening either pregnant women or infants for HIV are successful enough. It results into a drastic cut in further infection in our society when treatment with AZT (Zidovudine) has been good enough for pregnant women. Is it ethical to make such test compulsory for all pregnant women? Does such test violate her rights, liberties and privacy though she may not be careless about sex-behaviour? Is it not true that if infected women got good results, sane-head non-infected women should go for the same? These are questions which we do not merely put to pregnant women and her associates and acquaintances, but to the doctors, nurses and in house caretakers who are responsible in any maternity clinic or wards. These questions may be emotionally hazardous to us once we ask for HIV positive tests for fetus or at an appropriate neo-natal state when some effective treatment is available or, else the fetus may be eliminated for greater risks of life – even new-born may be eliminated. These are also queer moral questions for our medical fraternity, which better we do not skip because it is a bad habit in medical parlance. All these questions transcend time and locale but not completely because many clinical tests, researches and subsequent treatments should address to the conditions of the poor third world countries, the economic affordability and viability. Better, one should talk a lot about the education of the ethic of safe sex behaviour and many ethical-spiritual measures of self-control and behaviour management. The time has arrived at our part of the world and perhaps globally to find the *ethic of alternative public health care management* when AIDS comes to be a threat to our caretakers.

A few words now about caring for the disabled and the helpless before we consider our way to resolve these issues through dialogue. The terms "disabled" and "helpless" both stand for ethical scrutiny because in many recent writings rather than simplicity, brevity and economy of use, we prefer some respectable or dignified words towards very respectable people living in civil states. I am not very sure about the use of some terms making people more or less respectable or dignified but some deliberate use of terms are insulting, derogatory and without a human face. Hence, some people feel that "disabled", "crippled" and "handicapped" are some insulting ways or less respectable ways to use for denoting the physically and the mentally challenged people having some freedom, goodwill and rights as unchallenged people have. In fact, we may have a lively debate of the ethic of linguistic use here, which may not have far reaching effects on medical usage, but who knows that the emotive charges flowing within human sensitivity will not change ways of speaking and writing in bioscience at the cost of some uneconomic words. Nevertheless, I have personally no emotional crisis in using "disabled" and "helpless" along with lengthy "physically and mentally challenged" and "orphans and street dwellers" because greater ethicality lies in meeting such people with love and doing earnestly something than using fabulous words though nothing is wrong if fabulous usages accompany great thinking and doing. Ethics is not only about ethics of language use, it is something more. Taking this finely carved out liberty for me I would like to find out at the outset what "disabled" and "physically and mentally challenged" amounts to and the ethical questions that arise out of caring these people. The words "orphans" and "street dwellers" do not pose much problem for meaning clarification though they stand good ground for an ethical scrutiny of care. These people who may be economically called "helpless" does call for some meaning clarification as "helpless" itself does not convey the sense of "only the orphans and the street-dwellers". There are many practical and poetic ways to explain "helpless". One way is to explain my helplessness to strictly define "disabled" and "helpless". However, I shall try to explain the import of the notions along with their ethical overtones.

Disability is such a physical and mental state of a person which is rationally implausible to desire as such, rather, it is desirable that we are better not in such states because it is essentially "harmful" to body and mind. The physically and the mentally disabled or handicapped or challenged as we say, are thus people who are in some such states of body and mind, which are undesirable to them and they would desire they were not in such states or, in case they were to live with it, they should be *appropriately equipped* to face the challenge. This need for appropriate equipment calls for care, some cure if possible and some means for *adjustments to adversities*. All these things, care, cure and adjustments are needed from "outside" sources and from "within" because "internal" equipments are sources of facing negative harms on body and mind. It is well known that crippling disabilities have been won by people from "within" as supported from "outside", which is true of prolonged mental disabilities. Disabilities or challenges come to the caretakers in different forms, some of them needing emergent care from outside as the inner energy of the person does not function owing to unconscious or coma states as found in multiple injuries after severe road accidents. Whereas some others need systematic rational self-management immediately with some external aid or suggestion or guidance as in case of paralytic attacks or spinal injury. Caretakers are thus challenged with several physically and mentally disabled people who need *reversal* of situations prevailing or as in cases of business, speech and auditory handicap and other cases of a likely non-reversal of present conditions, should strive for *betterment*, more and more *empowerment*, *research* for a likely *partial or complete reversal*, *counselling* and *suggestions*. The explanation provided above might successfully cover some disabilities of gametes, embryos, fetus and neonates, all of which ask for some reversal of prevailing conditions of harm either partially or fully.

Once our caretakers are faced with the challenge of "reversal" of disabled conditions, as I have hinted before, many ethical questions creep in. Two extremely important questions pertain to "discrimination"; they are, why it should be ethically preferable to benefit or care a disabled rather than a non-disabled? And, what is ethically good in producing (or allowing) a disabled person to exist at the cost of troubling the non-disabled? The first takes us for many socially, economically and politically charged questions as well, all of them bearing some sense of ethical ought and right. The second takes us to more trifles like abortion, assisted killing and their ethical implications. Here we shall not go into the different replies collected in the bioethical literature because our method is different. Here is some food for thought to find out what ethical questions amount to with regard to cases of disability and why an ethic of care or medical care ethics are dragged to reply them. In one sense attending to these questions, we can find out the relevance of such ethical talk. Equally true is that we can justify why in public health care system it would not be more ethical to propagate the notion of "no care" than "some care" and why in such system careless attitude leading to disability should be aptly treated for reversal if not suggesting termination of life. John Harris puts it nicely: "Disability is somehow disabling and therefore undesirable. If it were not, there would be no motive to try to cure or obviate disability in health care more generally. If we believe medical science should try to cure disability where possible and that parents would be wrong to withhold from their disabled children's cures as they become available".[6] It is interesting to notice here that ethical questions of care of physically and mentally challenged people are no less important than those of the care of HRGs which, we have seen before. A comparison of both groups for relative importance of care would be in bad taste. However, the magnitude of the HRG care at this point of history makes a tough choice before health caretakers and the public in general; do we need more health care allocation and also health care professionals to combat the cases of HRGs than the other disabled persons? What should be the ethical course of action in this regard? Moreover, are we not facing a new set of challenges from the HRGs who make a unique group of physically and mentally disabled in our society? Is it true that our biomedical conception of the "handicapped" or "challenged people" should be reviewed in the light of the contemporary menace of AIDS in particular? The question is crucial when some AIDS victims are non-offenders in sexual habits and perversions. Equally important is to find out whether or not the notion of "helpless" should extend in view of such cases and not restrict it to the realm of orphans and street dwellers. It is interesting to notice that in India, the biomedical notion of the "helpless" should have changed phenomenally as we have been combating the vices of *thrown-out* physically challenged lepers and the mentally sick people, those who are living a life of either beggars or street people or a jailed life in asylums for they do not have any takers in society. Are they street dwellers? Are they free? Are AIDS victims not thrown-out, equally challenged for adoption, care and management? We may carefully think and find why HRGs, disabled and helpless together constitute a queer group asking different ethical questions of care. I think that these questions cannot and need not be answered by a thinker, a philosopher, a social activist, a doctor, a nurse or others in isolation. I do not have faith (as many others have) that such questions should be aptly faced by some "experts" in this field by applying their ethical knowledge of "four principles" or absolutely valid "ethical theories" or a combination of the two or by discussing human virtues and values. These are to me "artificial" ways to counter the above ethical dilemmas. Let us, therefore, have a glimpse of what I call "intersubjective corroboration", a method of resolving moral crises in health care.

Interestingly, in the mean time we have had sufficient introduction to the "problem in consideration" which, on the one hand focuses the theoretical-technical aspects of the problem in a not so technical manner for a number of readers not likely to follow the intricacies of biology and medicine, and on the other hand it brings out the possibility of ethics-talk about such problems along with a number of ethically charged questions for our perusal. The introduction also focuses our inclination to theory and/or principle cooption, as well as virtue and/or value cooption in answering the ethical questions. Such introduction also needs to stress on the typical Indian setting in which we are posed to resolve these ethical issues because without it, an ethics-talk is rather blank; we do not come to know what exactly we are talking about, why and in which social, political and economic contexts. Next step is to *select parties* for a moral dialogue and *framing questionnaire* which is immensely helped by the information one gets from an introduction like this one or a more rich deeper study of relevant literature and case studies. Further we come to the *conduction* of the *dialogue* and the *consensus* evolved with regard to the resolution of the moral problem in consideration. Finally, an ethicist or a well trained person in ethics should analyze the entire dialogue (*post corroboration analysis*) so as to find out the dynamic of ethical principles and theories, and the virtues and values of people participating in ethical resolution in a non-artificial manner.

There are many problems in *selection of concerned parties* in a meaningful intersubjective corroboration dialogue particularly when we are concerned with bioethical problems like the problem of public health care. First problem is that the number of technical questions that arise in this field are unique to the physicians and the nurses, which are not equally efficiently understood and addressed to by others. Nevertheless, we cannot neglect these ordinary people completely, for their moral opinions matter for all practical purposes.

Hence, given the problem of the ethic of care, we ought to concentrate on physicians and nurses mainly and on other people to some extent at least. Second problem is that a number of experts within the fields of medicine and nursing should be included in case of the problem of care because we need to listen to those dealing with neonatal care (HRG), chest care (HRG), neuro care (HRG), general surgery (HRG), general medicine, AIDS and infectious and communicable diseases care (HRG), care of accident and burn cases in emergency wards (HRG) and the psychiatrists (disabled and helpless) and counsellors (disabled and helpless), those who care for the blind, deaf and dumb (disabled and helpless) and those who are associated to orphanage and adoption centre (helpless). Now if we go on asking a range of ethically charged questions to one person representing these groups of caretakers, moral dialogue will go on and on and a closure with consensus will not be in view easily. Hence, I suggest a pragmatic way to selcction of parties for dialogue. First, we have to take some pain to talk to as many experts as possible taking care of the HRG's disabled and the helpless to do the following: (A) Try to know the several technical/theoretical and practical aspects of the problem in consideration so that a precise questionnaire for moral dialogue could be constructed; (B) Try to evaluate the depth and extent of the theoretical, technical as well as moral opinions of the experts you talk to so that a careful selection of panelists for a dialogue is possible; (C) Try to understand how practical questions should be placed in the moral dialogue so that rather than a technical dialogue in biomedicine, it becomes predominantly moral. It is desirable that like a well selected panel for discussion, most pertinent ethical questions are put to the experts which are comfortably answered by our panelists. Here it is important to notice that in India, where biomedical ethic is at its neo-natal stage, ethicists or other able persons interested in resolution through corroboration of moral views need not construct too many technical ethical questions like those mentioned in our earlier discussion because hopefully many of our experts do not have an idea about "four principles" or "ethical theories" or "virtue ethics" or "value theories" and about other tricky questions involving normativism, non-normativism, relativism, anti-theoreticism and so on. It is better as beginners in this field to initiate moral dialogues with our experts on the basis of some such questions, answers to which would nicely bring out the conception of experts about ethical desirability, good, right, just, duty, obligation and decision-making rules having a human face. Gradually when in countries like India the creed of moral dialogue gains some popularity, acceptance among the public health caretakers and other groups grows, and when people know more and more about what the moral dialogues reveal in so far as *academic ethics* is concerned, only then do we need more technical-ethical questions for ethical discourses or else it is the vanity of ethicists. Putting very grave ethical questions would thus mar our effort now. Soon the readers will come to know why despite a number of ethical questions, moral problems raised by me in the introductory part of the discussions do not figure in the "questionnaire" I have framed for the moral dialogue. We will come to know why in most parts of the earlier discussion I was averse to the different answers provided by bioethicists of the USA, the UK, Canada and Australia. It is a kind of prejudice on the part of an Indian ethicist or whosoever to fall in a *structuralist* trap to read bioethical literature made available to us by those working outside the Indian context and frame ethical questions exactly in their ways. There is no greatness in putting some difficult ethical questions by reading these literatures. We should be free and wise to construct questions bringing out the best of our minds. As I have said, when the creed of bioethical dialogues grow more grave questions may be discussed. One may ask: what was the necessity then to fill the pages of this book with so many information and problems for Indian readers? First, is that among these questions some are of most general or universal nature, which most likely we need not skip in ethical dialogue in any social context. Second, this book gives an outline of ethics of care as well as inciting our minds to find out the extent and depth of the issues covered by this, hoping that if we find some time, we think for ourselves independent of the pressures of information gathered and dumped on us. Third, after a glimpse of moral dialogue to be considered shortly, the replies, the consensus and finally, analysis of the dialogue, we shall come to know that without being "morally conditioned" by any literature to a great extent, we are able to express some such ethical opinions which often care to answer the interesting questions in the same way or most nearly in the same way as many other well-read people have answered. We shall thus hopefully find out resolution to a number of issues raised by bioethicists at different points of time though not being extremely theory coopted. Hopefully, we shall find out some leanings to principle or principles or theory or theories or virtue and values in the course of moral dialogues but that will not be of an expert. It will not be funny but interesting to discover that what has been found in the bioethical literature is not alien to many non-philosophers who unfold their moral opinions without any "moral conditioning".

Coming to the *questionnaire* now, we cannot completely neglect the patients, his or her attendants, and members of family, friends and other sympathizers for their moral opinion and for that reason it should be easily understood and answered. However, most of the time the moral views of these people need not be gathered in a long gruelling debate with physicians and other experts. Their opinions are best gathered in an extremely non-formal way by attending physicians and other health caretakers who also take interest in ethical matters. Talking to these people is difficult but not impossible if some time is allowed for that. Some care should be given to express what they feel about the decisions taken in an earlier consensus of opinions and some respect should be shown for these people in moral matters though they may be very hesitant or shaky about all this. Again we need not follow an American or Canadian pattern in India where in government hospitals patients and their associates wait in long queues or possibly in herds, where a fight for adjustable bed of rags on floor is intense, where one small room is shared by three or four doctors each eagerly surrounded by patients at critical states with their associates and where touts roam for an easy access to treatment or allocation or so many other things. Here, in India we need not stand with questionnaires of "yes" / "no" type to be filled in by these notoriously neglected people. Here, we need not have an intellectual ethicist with his team waiting to grab one opportunity to ask them: 'well nice guy, what is desirable in kidney donation?' However, the *in-house people* can do some homework by asking the patients and their associates whether or not certain decisions taken are ethically acceptable to them or something needs more careful scrutiny. I believe this will take some time in India. Hence, readers need not wonder that in none of the dialogues I explained here, patients and associates are not directly involved. Yet, in some dialogues while framing questions and shaping decision-making rules, such people have been contacted by this author, about which we shall come to know at a proper place. There is no need of skepticism on the part of people interested in a social scientific venture like this one that talking to ailing people and associates is impossible. It is not impossible rather; it needs great effort, time and team-work including support from the in-house people. Maybe some of our interested medical or nursing students will take up this challenge or many ethicists come to face the music with people on ground realities of suffering and care. I must say that though lack of formal education is not a block to the success of moral discourse and resolution, the spread and acceptance of people's participation in bioethical matters at least demands some degree of infrastructural and allied uplift in medical care because such talk with people is possible at a stage of freedom from the daily pangs for basic care. But equally true is that to make this uplift possible, people should participate in full force so that their voice is heard. Hence, a complete lackadaisical boorish attitude towards education, rights and fight for rights do not enable bioethical discourse a complete success.

I will now state the questions framed by me for moral dialogue involving the following people. Mrs. C.K. Mariama, Retired Head Matron of Rajendra Medical College and Hospital, Ranchi; Dr. R.R. Bhattacharjee, Former CMO, H.E.C Hospital, Ranchi; Dr. S. Mukherjee, General Medicine, Specialist in Leprosy Care, Ranchi; Dr. S. Haque Nizami, Central Institute of Psychiatry, Ranchi; Dr. Alka Nizami, "Deep Shikha", Centre for caring the physically and mentally challenged children, Ranchi; Dr. Mithilesh Kanti, Former Principal, Netarhat School, Director, "Deep Shikha", Ranchi and Mrs. Dolly Punnoose and Mrs. James Punnoose with the children of the "Bethel Mission" Home for the helpless people, Ranchi.

QUESTIONNAIRE

1. What should be the ultimate goal of public health care that includes caring the high risk group of patients, the disabled and the helpless people in our society?
2. As health care professionals and concerned citizens how would you like to enlist your rights, duties and obligations towards the people of your society needing care?
3. Who do you think should be made accountable in a civil society towards public health care? How do you look into the goodness of an involvement and accountability of the non-government institutions and organizations *vis-à-vis* the government institution and organizations?
4. Do you think that "isolation" of one group of people needing care from other groups, such as isolating the high risk group from the helpless, the disabled and common people is ethically right or just?
5. How would you justify the ethicality of disparities in health

care allocation in our society keeping in view the necessity of "isolation" as well as imbalance in our purchase capacity of health care amenities?

6. What is ethical in "isolating" physically and mentally challenged people for education? How should such education function in this regard?
7. Is it morally just to empower the common people including ailing masses, the disabled and the helpless with knowledge of basic rights to live a good healthy life and the legal aspects involved in a neglected or wrong ways of treatment and care? How do you look into the aspects of consumerism and legality in this regard?
8. How would you justify the ethic of adoption of helpless people? Do you take it as a bargain? Do you think that selection progresses in adoption, particularly of orphans should be governed by sex, colour and genetic selection and adoption at a distance?
9. In the light of the consensus emerged in the discussion, what specific guidelines regarding public health care would you like to suggest?

A little reflection on the selection of the panelists and the questions would reveal that I was trying to be cautious about greater participation of concerned people, including the experts in this field and the non-structuralist questions that would cover the moral opinions regarding this matter to a large extent. In fact, if we ourselves do not get involved in one such discourse it is very difficult to show you how these people comfortably and extremely wisely replied these questions to bring out almost everything about the ethic of care, about which we have seen something in the introductory part. The participants, however, had no idea whatsoever of a number of questions I raised in the introduction but we will find answers to most of these trifling questions. Let us, therefore, read about what was revealed in the dialogue. I shall take up one panelist after another and then analyze the outcome of the dialogue.

Mrs. Mariama thinks that her long association in government hospital for public health care that percolates to the poorest of the poor has enabled her to realize that *the highest goal in health care is maximization of the physical and mental good of the public in general and the patients in particular*. She thinks that nothing could be said separately about the care of the high risk group of patients, the disabled and the helpless because ultimately for all of them we strive to give the best and most physical and mental well-being. She thinks that being a nurse and a responsible matron for a long time she is obliged to serve the nation selflessly by doing her bit of duty in an extremely professional and not amateurish way. She is aware of what her profession demands and what more she can do if needed. She is also aware of her right to create an atmosphere of discipline, cleanliness, regularity, punctuality, dedication and compassion that enhances speedy recovery of health. Mrs. Mariama is of the opinion that first and foremost, accountability in health care is of the health care professionals. Among them she feels that she herself is most accountable to her colleagues, doctors and patients. She is perhaps accountable even to the general public who need proper care at a time of distress or when they are in good health because one remains in good health when there is a back-up care. Secondly, the government who has been represented by our people is directly accountable to the good of the public in many ways, health care being one such way. Though government cannot do anything and everything for this vast population if the public themselves do not participate in maintaining good health and hygiene. She thinks that some private institutions and NGOs may be of use but that does not happen if they are only profit oriented. Health care cannot be made an exclusive business.

Mrs. Mariama thinks that isolating one group of people from another group is needed only at practical levels but at the theoretical level of care, there is no such need because all await their good. However, practically speaking, isolation is at times desirable just to achieve the higher goal in health care, so it is good for the people as well. Certainly, we need special methods to care for the AIDS patients, the severely handicapped people, very sick orphans and the neo-natal cases as they cannot be treated in the same method as we normally obtain. Once, the good of these people prevails, they come to know that they are not being neglected or that some people are scared of their state. We must keep in mind that health caretakers also have a precious life, which should be protected, otherwise their good will be neglected, which is again not good but evil. Mrs. Mariama holds that distinguishing one class of patients from another class for better care is not ethically good at all, though in government hospitals we do have paid accommodations for better comfort but that does not necessarily mean that better care has been given to them. If knowingly the doctors and the nurses give affluent people better care than the poor and needy residing in crowded general wards, it is essentially unethical because in doing so the good of much precious life is not possible. Similarly, if there is disparity in government allocation, that is, poor allocation in case of health care than more allocation in any other less vital sector, it is essentially unethical for human life is precious to a nation. Mrs. Mariama argues that separate methods of treating and educating physically and mentally handicapped people are ethical ideas for the reason stated before. She warns that if we are able to find a system to prevent quacks from treatment, only then participation of common people or those who are not well-trained in scientific ways may be valuable in a limited way because doing things amateurishly and in a wrong manner does more bad than good, and thus unethical. In cases of improper care, therefore, or neglect of duty, the patients have every moral right to sue a person legally because professional responsibility and rights are to do good and not bad. Mrs. Mariama thinks that adoption is not bargain; it should be done under strict government and public vigil. In any case it is ethical because it does some good to the helpless. According to Mrs. Mariama, today we are in need of more nursing training schools which impart good scientific training along with the teachings of moral and human values. She thinks that the government should be more concerned about raising health care standards in government hospitals because here care is for the needy mass who cannot afford costly treatment.

Dr. R.R. Bhattacharjee holds that the ethical goal of public health care is *overall betterment of the suffering people worldwide.* It is important to notice that in providing such care, the professionals also develop their own self through empathy. It is also important for him that an attitude which is truly professional takes health care as a noble service, as a social responsibility to help people in utter distress and to perform according to the professional demands in different conditions. Dr. Bhattacharjee thinks that non-interference, pity and sympathy are not preferable over the conceptions of equality and total involvement of the physicians in health care. A feeling of participation in suffering encourages a patient, he thinks. The sense of unity grows. He holds that empathy is not hindrance to medical professionalism, it is rather a booster to civil as well as ethical life because *the higher ideal is the holistic well-being of the person*, which is possible when you do not merely prescribe, rather counsel, share and enable the sufferer to get better in an efficient way. Dr. Bhattacharjee thinks that in practice the application of the theory of *Vedānta in medicine* may not be possible mechanically though the ideal of *nsṣkāma karma* of the *Gitā*, is possible even by ordinary people. He thinks that when it comes to health care it should be both individual and socially directed as well as both for the maximization of pleasure and holistic well being. The holistic care and holistic medical assistance needs these things. He believes that as a part of this, alternative methods of health care in India are very important such as *Yogic care and psychotherapies* by experts and other counsellors. For Dr. Bhattacharjee accountability on the part of the physicians is extremely important for it is ethical. It helps in achieving the highest goal in health care. Every lay person thus has the right to know what is going on in treatment, what are the do's and don'ts, what are the chances of recovery and what is the present status. Without such knowledge, a civil society lacks a proper health care management. About talking truth to AIDS or other patients he thinks that it is a part of social education, it is a must for the greater good, without much worrying about its evil use by a crooked person. He thinks that though in practice doctors need to get results, they use placebos on ethical grounds though that may be concealing some truth. A doctor needs to be good therapist and a counselor not just one who prescribes lengthy medicines. In India, both public and private sector participation is needed in health care. More needed is participation of some sane heads helping people at grassroots level. Equally true is that doctors should go to the villages and to the poorest of the poor for care.

Mr. James and Mrs. Dolly Punnoose shared their views by saying that the ethic of care is based on the Love to the neglected and needy. Love is the element of goodness as given by God and inherent in our nature which we want to share while we care. This is not doing drab duty or fulfilling obligation or having own happiness or extending happiness to all. It is the simple notion of love spreading it from self to others. However, one who does not have any regard for the truth that God is represented as love cannot feel to have achieved that goal through care. This way if we live our life of help and care to realize the ideal of universal love, we say, we come closer to the realization of God. Hence, care in one way attains realization of God in us.

Mrs. Dolly says that you see something special in a child, not as a subject or an object or a commodity or even the one who depends on us rather as godly a creation of God, and as such, epitome of Love.

Love spreads through creation and when we care, a child, it is love that is connected among humans.

Mrs. James holds that in so far as the atheists are concerned, surely they do not take child as embodiment of God or do not take us as creation of God, they may still participate in caring the child who is helpless but may be because they do it as a professional duty or a social good or that it is good for him or her. However, to us, care does not mean anything like this; it is nothing but expression of love or God within us. Morally speaking, for us a Marxist would have a political project while caring a helpless which is repugnant to us because we do not think that the goal of care is to achieve some political agenda. We care for we love or want to spread love. We care because God loves creations selflessly. Mrs. Dolly adds that her helpless children needs both sympathy and empathy because loving them would need both on our part. We need to have sympathy owing to their neglected condition and empathy for we need to identify ourselves to their horrid conditions – we need to feel 'One' in care. She argues that we do not think that any amount of self-satisfaction overwhelms the elements of self-sacrifice, sympathy and empathy in health care or care for the disabled and helpless people. Hence, self-satisfaction is never the end of care though great degree of self-sacrifice is needed in care, which is again great but not for self benefit or self-esteem. If we keep these things in mind with the ideal of love as supreme, we must accept the truth that we support the "matriarchic" pattern of care than the "patriarchic" care in this patriarchic Indian society. Care is never at best at a distance, as a professional duty, as obligation, as happiness and as self-satisfaction – it is care like a patriarch not an empathetic, all loving mother. Caring is thus not a business; it is an involvement of self with God.

Both James and Dolly Punnoose think that it is not necessary to train helpless and disabled people for their political rights and their legible demands as much as they need true education that enable them to stand on their own, have freedom, think independently and above all, learn the goodness of God and Love so that they contribute towards spreading love in the universe. True care leads to ethical man-making not a political man-making. Both the Punnoose thus hold that special reservations and isolations for the helpless and the handicapped at every sphere of public life is not ethically desirable because fixing a reservation counter or some seats in trains and buses do not make them feel any better or worse. What we need more is striving for equal status and better empowerment of these people in social life. The Punnoose think that the idea of segregated schooling and training of disabled and helpless, particularly the deaf, dumb and blind as well the idea of such schools completely cut off from mainstream schools is not ethically desirable as the element of human bond in love is absent. We need more and more mainstream schools opening out for methods of teaching where special instructors work and the children stay and learn with other non-challenged students. Punnoose think that their Bethel Town is also a school where orphans stay and study with others who come from different families. Here children know that they live in hostel and not in an orphanage. Even the idea of a 'Home for orphanage' is an ethically unacceptable idea to them because that divides us from within.

Mr. James thinks that though equality of opportunity in educational empowerment is ethically desirable, given the economic status of Indians and the state of governance here, the best people to impart such empowerment are the NGOs and the private institutions because they have the right to do things as Churches did to enable many disabled and helpless people attain good positions. Yet, if the government does not adequately support, the legal system does not back up and financial flow is not smooth, such social objectives are difficult to attain.

Both argued about "adoption" that it is always an ethically good choice than ultramodern ways to have babies like we are having test tube babies. In India and many other places these things are far from easy and accessible. It would be more good, think many, to live ever in friction in a family by not having a child or a test-tube baby than sharing and caring with one who is not yours but becomes one with you in love. Our parenthood is fulfilled through this selfless love in adoption. Both felt that in adoption a child is not a commodity and adoptors are not bargainers though many take it like that or some might earn from the bargain. To Mr. and Mrs. Punnoose, where love is the motto, adoption is not a bargain, though at times, legality prevents from adoption as they themselves were prevented from adopting one child when they had two daughters but now their pursuance has led to a Town of sixty adopted children.

Both James and Dolly are empathetic in rejecting all sorts of health check-ups even at the risk of selecting HIV infected child for adoption if true love rules supreme in this matter. You just cannot select creations on the basis of sex, colour and health status they argued. Even if we are natural parents and our child picks up Hepatitis B, we risk our lives for her care. Similarly, we should go for adoption what may come to us. If after adoption we find some grave malady, we shall collectively fight for its removal and not give up. Both the participants said that participation of government agencies, the government hospitals and free treatment by doctors of the helpless, disabled and very poor people is desirable but we expect more involvement of private benevolence on the part of doctors and lay people trained in basic health care to come to us for help. This includes teaching these children and even counselling free of cost. These ideas are good for the welfare of poor people as well. Donations in this regard from any agency are also good.

Dr. Siddhartha Mukherjee thinks that Public Health Care includes care for the healthy people and not only the sick ones. In India, unlike many countries where government takes care of 90 percent of the public health care seriously, something has gone wrong. Here people come to hospitals and to the private doctors when they are sick or else there is little care for the general mass consisting of the disabled and the helpless for good healthy life and not merely for sickness. The ultimate goal of health care is thus *holistic biological well-being of the masses of nations without any discrimination for status, caste, class etc. and well followed up by adequate empowerment of disabled and helpless to live a dignified human life.* So far the question of rights, duties and obligation are concerned, the health care professionals do enjoy unique rights to holistic well-being as empowered by their training, the oath of service and the institutional rules. Duties and obligations the health care experts have are immense as they are morally bound to the society as responsible social beings to serve human kind impartially and benevolently. It is needed on their part to ever transcend their fixed duties and obligations to sick people to help them by providing free treatment and medicines if needed. Unless some care is taken for such benevolence, health care is not possible. He thinks that the doctors, the nurses and many NGOs, who are serious in public health care, should have close liaison among them for free treatment to the needy, helpless and disabled for without any social compassion and faith in unity of mankind, ideal of health care is not attainable. Health care is not all about making money or making good healthy conditions of living at the expenditure of good money. Dr. Mukherjee thinks that being a follower of Sri Rāmakrishṇa Paramhmasa, according to his *Vedāntic* ideal, he prefers sympathy and empathy but not pity and pleasure as means to the realization of holistic biological well-being because sympathy and empathy are elements related to realization of unity of mankind – basic "oneness" among us so to say. Hence, if we are able to treat humanity as ourselves or as divine selves so to say, then in that way we are successful in realization of the health care ideal. It is not true that the realization of the ideal gives us pleasure or happiness because more than that, holistic well-being is much greater idea. It is closer to our ability of realization of the Higher Self. Health care is one way in realizing the ideal of oneness of Self, we may say. However, it is not true that those who do not adhere to this ideal are not care takers, rather, they may be still striving for the ideal of health care, that is, the biological well-being. Hence, for all practical reasons putting a condition that biological well-being is possible only when we realize Divine Self will be demanding too much in a complex society. It would be equally ethical for an atheist who strives for the public health care as driven by the ideals of selfless care, benevolence, sympathy and empathy. So far as the question of physicians dealing with patients and families is concerned, though these days physicians have less time, they are expected to talk to the patients as friends, as counsellor and as ones who tell a truth if needed about seriousness of his or her disease and about personal hygiene because they are related to social hygiene as well. For uneducated people some necessary truth is needed for a sure and safe cure. Some taboos and dogmas need firm dealing when we take social value of public health care. Most important for health caretakers is to see the ailing people of all categories as very important as one's own self or, better said, where equanimity of view is a way of life, where treatment is not a passion or a means to earn. Without this way of life, a health caretaker cannot ethically justify his actions. In India one who has no care for the economic status of the poor, and strives for public welfare, the person cannot ethically attain his goal in life. This is more prominent when we come to treatment of leprosy with which more social misconceptions and taboos are related than truth. Here, we need no segregation but equal treatment. We need to approach them as people who are likely to be cured and not cursed. The risk is high in some cases of infection but we can segregate them temporarily and not permanently for that creates a rift and not love and unity. Dr. Mukherjee thinks that in the MBBS courses adequate introduction to the ethic of public health care and methods of counselling are necessary. More on education, he thinks that in books of health and hygiene we need to introduce what diseases are of high risk and the way we ought to approach these patients with dignity. Coming to the problem of the ethic of adoption, Dr. Mukherjee thinks that selections on the basis of race, caste, colour is unethical as that is against the ideal of oneness. It is equally unethical to not to adopt a high risk child as one suffering from thalassaemia because one has to strive for the child's well-being when one adopts and not shy away from it. On the same ground, sex selection in adoption is unethical. Legal intervention is necessary in adoption but rules preventing wrong selections are needed. In any case adoption and infertility need not be necessarily related. If one likes to adopt children, to them, the matter of infertility should come secondary. Dr. Mukherjee finally stressed that in our country more cooperation among the government and non-government organizations are needed in public health care with sufficient budgetary allocation.

Dr. S. Haque Nizami and Dr. Alka Nizami both emphasized that they are non-believers, though they do not have anything against the believers. Hence, for them the question of monotheism as the basis of ethicality and the basis of health care practices does not make much sense. Science being secular, it is the best healer of mankind and their suffering without any favour. Healing is thus based on a secular discipline called science and the ethic of healing needs that we have faith on secular science and not on any taboo or faith or religious doctrine. Dr. S.H. Nizami adds that the state of health care rights and government allocation towards public health care are in unsatisfactory states since the initiation of our planning and budgetary allocation. Population growth and lack of proper education leads to ignorance about health care rights, how to get those rights, how to seek justice and how to strive for better allocation. The clear unethicality of a poor system of allocation is that it does not do enough *welfare of the masses*, which is so needed. The main reason behind the crunch situation in public health care by the government as could be seen in our Sadar Hospitals and medical college and hospitals is owing to poor infrastructure and management largely based on poor allocation as well as poor use of funds. Several malpractices make things worse. It would not be a poor idea, therefore, that even if the utilitarian and the welfaristic ideals have their own problems, they are nevertheless desirable in our context lest some private sector is made accountable to contribute to the welfare of the public by improving health conditions. It is not a matter of competition between the public and the private sectors, it is a matter of accountability, says Dr. Alka Nizami. On the part of the private sector to do some business, having profits is good but an imperative should be there to contribute to health care of the population with whom they work and earn. It is ethically desirable, therefore, that we have more private participation in the management of the public hospitals. This would need some degree of autonomy and privilege on the part of the private houses though government rules and checks always act as deterrence. There is no doubt that the business houses in health care should get exemptions and cuts when it comes to substantive contribution to the public health care, which, however, is not care of a section but participation in mass care. The state of private participation in Indian health scenario is guided by a welfaristic ideal as this is a welfare state. These houses should be made accountable if needed by law towards public health care and education. Equally true is that our government institutions cannot avoid the idea of self-sustenance if any more subsidy or greater budgetary allocation proportionate to population is not in view. Relative autonomy of government institutions for raising funds by providing paid care to some sectors cannot be completely neglected. If these things are not there, the state of the health care of the poor will be in bad shape, which is grossly unethical if *welfarism is the ideal*. Dr. A. Nizami says even the small NGOs who work for better public health care must first have some earnest will to achieve an ideal and then they have to do some really hard work to raise funds and to campaign. It is not that the NGOs cannot maximize good for the people. In fact, with egoism and profit making motives alone, no NGO, private and public institution can be successful in the long run in health care.

Dr. A. Nizami thinks that when NGOs or others appeal to the common people or a business house for funds to care for the helpless and the disabled, they do everything out of pity and sympathy because they are least involved in the pain and suffering of the needy people. However, empathy should be ethically speaking the motive of public health care on the part of the physicians, NGOs, nurses and so on or else they are not one with those who need care. Dr. Nizami agrees that though maximization of happiness of the people through holistic health care is their objective, they do not find health care professionals, doing their duty for the sake of duty as anything noble because their professional duty aims at the biological welfare, which is supreme. Equally true is that though monotheistic ethics has no value for them, they would prefer liberal ethics more than any other theory because a professional performance of duty for *biological well-being amounts to self-satisfaction as well.* A person gets some amount of freedom to do his duties in the best way available to him and he gets satisfied when he does so. Hence, 'care is only social-directed', is not a good idea because the feeling of the caretaker that one is doing something great for someone is less valuable than the conception that the care taker is not helping or doing a great favour or even is a selfless person, rather he is striving for a health care objective to fulfil his or her professional excellence or to satisfy himself or herself as a professional. The doctors think that in health care practice egoism (non-hedonistic type) has its own value, as valuable as utilitarianism and welfarism, though the conception of duty for duty is less important for them in comparison to ethical egoism, which theory they believe, has been underestimated. But in health care, particularly in mental health care, one can never visualize a position when your intervention would amount to definite return. Hence, the point of gains or returns does not become important in the face of professional performance of duty, though self-satisfaction and self-fulfilment does matter. Dr. S. Haque Nizami thinks that in public health care one crucial aspect is right to information apart from right to care which is related to 'right to know'. But the health caretaker needs to be judicious. Ethically speaking, if the person has a contagious or a non-contagious illness which is fatal or that the person is terminally ill, we have to evaluate where right to information and knowing truth holds good and physicians should divulge it or provide it. This is needed for the social good; the welfare of social health is equally important as personal health, and in cases like AIDS or highly contagious diseases the truth has to be told to the patient or to the attendants so that they act likewise. Dr. Alka Nizami thinks that in cases like AIDS the person not only has to be told the truth, he has to be educated in personal and social hygiene as well as the person needs segregation whether you prefer egoism or utilitarianism or welfarism. However, history of segregation tells us that we have been constantly changing our ways in health care in this regard owing to medical inventions. Hence, segregation of leprosy and epileptic patients are no more ethical because the good of those who contribute to the society is not in view.

Dr. Nizami argues that the very concept of segregation does not apply to mentally handicapped children any more for the same ethical reason because today in the field of education we have specially equipped schools with special educators who teach them along with other children. Parallel, however, we have special schools which need not assume the form of a segregated place. The concept of mental health care with no boundaries is spreading therefore. The concept of integrated edncation has problems. One is regarding the integration of severely retarded children through education. These children need most care for a long duration and to negotiate them, special schools are not the right place. The normal schools should open out to accommodate them by having special wings for them. There are infrastructural and financial facilities which "Deepshikha" does not have as compared to them. What is then missing in our normal schools is the motivation and the ethical urge to do well, which, with all adversities small institutions like "Deepshikha" have. In any case isolating children is not an ethical idea in schools. In so far as having strict government intervention through legislation is a fabulous idea lest it does not boomerang for what is crucial is not legislation but the ethic of care which is the basis to motivate us to integrate through education. Hence, any imperative or flow of funds does not make integration possible. Dr. A. Nizami tells us that the ethical basis of integrated health care as such is flourishing human welfare or optimum welfare of humans. This ideal is not against the utilitarian ideal as well as the liberal or individualistic ethical ideal because here we are speaking of both personal good, personal happiness and also social good and social happiness.

Dr. Nizami thinks that community health care is a missing notion in India particularly when it comes to the care of the mentally challenged people because as members of a community these people have been thoroughly neglected since a long time by the government and by the people of our nation. The stigma of insanity prevented sane people to neglect and to segregate them than integrate in the whole. The paucity of mental health caretakers, particularly the psychotherapist and the counsellors are so much that we need to seriously think about educating common people about community care and about caring the mentally challenged. May be for this, in the education system or in special arrangements we train people as efficient psychotherapists. Another point is about the ethic of the physicians to act as bosses or jailors but not empathizers in mental health care. In community care, particularly when we speak of caring the mentally challenged ones, any person assuming supremacy and jailor attitude is unethical for it is against the sick individual's autonomy. If there is no regard or respect for individuality and autonomy, perhaps health care is a misnomer.

Dr. A. Nizami believes that sanctions of doctors have to be there and it necessarily does not amount to a jailor mentality because too much of liberalism as in USA (in this respect), is ridiculous. The experience in India is much better because here despite individuality, respect and autonomy, we still believe that some sanction has to be there if some good for the sufferer is to be achieved. Hence, rather than complete liberalism, we should better think for the social good in this respect and then it comes to imposition of care-codes on reluctant receivers of care. Dr. Nizami holds that when it comes to the question of religious counselling or religious based psychotherapy, though India, being religiously permeated country, it may not be an ethical idea at all to adopt it in our secular health care institutions though in our institutions we need to evaluate the different value systems of the patients and for that purpose questions about faiths are asked but that does not amount to religiously motivated therapy. Nor do we suggest the family members to do anything like that when it comes to the person's care in the community. The basic ethical reason is that religious beliefs have nothing to do with the betterment of the persons' good or welfare, though medical science does have many proven things to do for his or her good.

Mr. Mithilesh Kanti says that the ultimate goal of health care in general and the mental health care of the children in particular is complete physical and mental well-being of the person who is either sick or who is healthy. The good for the public is sound health, enjoyable life and flourishing of character. The obligations of health caretakers are to assure such things in society so that people remain valuable contributors in our societies. He thinks that basically health care is an individual effort of a physician or a nurse or others and it is satisfaction of the self by performing one's professional obligations properly which motivates the caretaker to persist in that service. However, individuals make society, and the social beings or the collective too have certain social obligations towards the sick people, which need not be neglected. This is more important in mental health care. In fact, the professional health caretaker is more concerned about the individual care primarily and about social well-being secondarily. Hence, his obligation is both individual and social directed. Mr. Kanti is emphatic that though the aim of public health care is well-being of individuals of societies, we cannot avoid the ethical value of non-hedonic or refined ethical egoism as motivating theory towards attaining the goal because in maximizing good for others we have no moral right to say that we have no care for the pleasure and satisfaction we get from treating a terminally and a mentally retarded child.

Sometimes this ideal seems to conflict with the ideal of pleasures for others, but it is not so because the physicians or others do not contest altruism, they are altruistic but do not disregard egoism. Further, when it comes to care of the mentally retarded, those who are expected not to recognize your service the other day, those who do not return anything, and you selflessly care them, you are not gross hedonic egoist or a psychological egoist rather an altruist – a welfarist. You really become *"nirahamkāri"*, that is, free from self-esteem and pride. Mr. Kanti thinks that on the basis of his support of egoism, he would not like to propagate an exclusive idea of empathy and oneness or unification of selves etc. in health care. He thinks that a mixed feeling of pity giving way to sympathy and satisfaction of helping are undeniable. Most of us who do not have any feeling of sympathy or oneness are equally ethical when we care for the high risk group of people, the disabled and the helpless. Empathy in reality might take away the objectivity of health care because the physician, caring a sick, has to essentially differentiate him in suggesting, prescribing, rebuking, sanctioning, using psychotherapies for greater good which is not possible with the sense of empathy and oneness. Mr. Kanti was unambiguous in rejecting monotheistic ethics of *Vedānta* as well as the Kantian and the *Gitā* type of deontology as theories guiding health care because the ultimate goal as he says is altruistic – welfare so to say in which permeates our pleasures and satisfaction. Hence, there is no scope for health care profession to skip the natural conclusion that in the name of duty or oneness or empathy we aim at maximization of our pleasure and nothing more than that, and truly this is ethical as nothing evil could be seen in both human welfare and having satisfaction. Mr. Kanti holds that right to information about health care is justifiable keeping in mind the ethical ideal he proposes. In fact, all of us should know about the legal aspect related to health care and about our right to sue wrong doers. Some kind of counselling, preaching and training is needed regarding this matter in our society when it comes to telling stark truth. Mr. Kanti says that it is a necessity but to be divulged with care and precision to the patients and/or the attendants so that greater good is not harmed. This is needed particularly in case of highly contagious diseases and fatal ones like AIDS. There is no point in thinking that truth is not needed at times. It is needed, not in bare nakedness but artfully. Coming to the question of giving rights and privileges to the handicapped people and their segregation as well as education Mr. Kanti thinks that nothing is unethical in giving them a different status, rights and privileges because they and normal people should know that everybody does not enjoy same privileges, capacities, powers etc. for many natural or unnatural reasons. It is due to the welfare of these people that distinction and segregation are needed though greater responsibility is on the normal people because they have to open out to help these people. This is true of educating the helpless and the handicapped as well. The pitiable situation of education of the disabled in mainstream schools mainly owes to lack of the ethic of care and some kind of supremacy that rules the psyche of the normal people. The truth is that handicapped people themselves are very good students and teachers. It is a pity not to see these people in our educational institutions. Rather, we find them at particular work places as if some stigma goes with them. Holistic welfare is not possible this way. About health care allocation and involvement of government sector in health care, Mr. Kanti is sceptical because he thinks that our government has perhaps run out of time, money and all wits to allocate more in the public health care; much now depends on the participation of the private sector though the moral scrutiny and checks on their activities are needed as well. He thinks that in India greater involvement of ordinary people in health care at the grassroots level and the role of the bare foot doctors and counsellors have become dire necessities for which they need some training. Mr. Kanti emphasizes that so much ignorance about caring mentally and physically challenged is that people do not know where to go and what to do. They are thus more often exploited by general physicians or they are prevented from going to a mental hospitals or a psychiatrist. These things will change only through education.

Keeping all these things in mind, after the lengthy discourse was over and a number of inquiries made, the corroborator ethicist drew the following points as *part* of a profound body of decision-making rules in health care in India, which has been derived out of not merely theoretical and practical but ethical scrutiny. Let us have a glimpse of these rules along with an idea of what has been corroborated on ethical lines and then I shall consider the final task of *post-corroboration analysis* of the discourse which is specific ethical task mostly undertaken by ethicists. The broad consensus available about the *ultimate end* of health care is to state simply: "Biological well-being of the global citizens". Biological well-being covers both physical and mental well-being which sidesteps further complexities about a race or a nation and wholesome well-being in terms of spiritual, metaphysical and transcendental well-being. The elements of development of character, flourishing of self, self-realization and fulfilment, all have been successfully avoided. This is possible if we carefully go through the views expressed here and by virtue of larger acceptance among the participants that after all public *health care* though related to a person as a whole, does not take too much burden on assurance of what has been nicely portrayed about a person. This was particularly needed when our participants, consisting of staunch believers, non-believers and secularists came to realize that *rationally speaking* professionals in public health care *ethically* target at achieving one specific goal that is desirable, and not too many things at one time though there is no doubt that what we call human good or overall human "welfare" is not merely "biological welfare", it is something more; but once to enter into "something more" there are problems. Hence, in case of medicine, the sensible objective is "holistic biological welfare". An ethically dormant person or the one who has no care for ethical scrutiny or we may say the one not ethically conscious about public health care, does not aim at the biological good of people worldwide. There are no stiff disagreements among our participants in accepting further that the ethical obligation of the health care professionals is, therefore, "assurance of the physical and mental good of the public who are presently not ailing from a disease or those who are sick needing immediate attention". The *duty* of the health care professionals, therefore, as stated by our participants is, "performing according to their professional expertise, codes and rules to their best of knowledge and ability for attaining the health care objectives being motivated by the spirits of sympathy, compassion and satisfaction of the professional-self". The *rights* of the health care professionals as gathered from the consensus is, "social, moral, professional and legal wherein the health caretakers enjoy the right of doing good for humanity at large and thus good for social health, cure and eradication of diseases as far as possible, to use the professional know-how and technical expertise as efficiently as possible without any ulterior objective than the basic health care objective, to have moral authority to enter into scrutiny of the ought and the good of all professional decision-making and respect the given legal binding of a state within professional activity and when necessary strive for accommodation of fresh sets of legal rights and to abolish some redundant or unethical ones. This further includes right to divulge truth, get information and to give information, to ask for declaration when needed and to get access to necessary aids and methods as and when deemed to be essential".

The corroboration further crystallizes *accountability* in health care in terms of the "individual and the collective". "All health care professionals and sub-professionals including the NGOs and the grass-roots health workers are accountable to the biological good of the people of a nation to which they belong primarily and to the humanity and the living world at large. The governments of all nations are accountable to public health care to great extent in allocating resources, funds, infrastructure, to construct legal bindings for several checks in the field and to efficiently implement them. They are expected to provide special financial facilities as per the needs and economic status of the larger whole without profit motive. The private houses doing business in health care as well as in other fields are expected to substantially contribute to the biological well-being of the people of the nation where they work and derive profit. The profit motive in the business of health care cannot be beyond legal rules of a state, cannot be unethical and exploitative. The profit accrued should be reasonably shared for the public health care".

It has been agreed to state that for all practical purposes in public health care, we should have effective and safe methods of *isolating* high risk group of patients, the highly contagious cases as well as the severe cases of mental deformities and disabilities for special care. However, there should be systematic *abolition* of all unnecessary isolations of patients in the mainstreams of national life. This is needed in case of the disabled and the helpless as well. Better ways to accommodate these people in the mainstream through enough empowerment is ethically desirable. It has been urged in the consensus about health care *allocation* that "no disparity is ethically viable and practically needed in civil states regarding health care on the basis of colour, race, caste, creed, sex and on the basis of difference of income or power to purchase care. This last criterion for allocation holds good in Indian context today though the private houses are not legally bound to do that though on high grounds of morality they should take care or a large number of the economically underpowered people".

Regarding *education* of the physically and mentally challenged children and the helpless ones, the consensus reveals that "the government is morally, socially, politically and legally bound to educate all sections of people of all age groups without any discrimination, and for that substantive funds for special instruction schools (also instructors) are needed in the mainstream schools run by government and private institutions. Thus, to reserve seats for the handicapped and the helpless is insufficient; they should have special wings to accommodate these people in a method of complete integration through learning so that the concept of special school or segregated learning is gradually abolished. The private institutions should be morally accountable to do so and if needed, should be legally compelled to do the same at a reasonable level. In cases of lack of financial support, these institutions should give certain scholarships or fee-cuts and government or other agencies should appropriately support them".

About *adoption*, the panel concluded that "the existing laws of adoption should take care of selections of sex, colour and genetics if that is gradually prevailing in our society or elsewhere because these being unethical, need to be prevented, though medical check-ups before selection cannot be ethically ruled out as for the biological good of the child, it may be needed for cure and care. It would be however a matter of voluntary choice that the sick or the one having fatal contagious disease may be closely monitored".

Most earnestly the participants believed that though the consensus after moral debate has resulted into the statements made here, we may still point out several finer points in the shape of desirable rules for our professionals. Statement of some of these points are needed even though in the above report of consensus are inherent some extremely important decision-making rules which need thorough scrutiny and clear formulation. Here are some rules:

Autonomy of health care professionals such as nurses in enforcing an atmosphere of proper health care through discipline, punctuality. cleanliness, regularity and dedication, the lack of which need to be stringently dealt within government hospitals in particular without favour, malice and pressure of the peer groups. (Mariama)

Rather than being louder about accountability of others, one should be more accountable first in public health care. It would need some reasonable degree of extra duties to be performed not necessarily mechanical following or rules. (Mariama)

Adequate safeguards of the lives of the health care professionals need to be assured at their work places. (Mariama)

Quacks and untrained nurses, midwifes and others need to be prevented from health care. Grassroots health caretakers should be trained and need to be reasonably used as and when we need them most. (Mariama and Bhattacharjee)

More nursing training schools with knowledge of advanced techniques and ethic of care are needed. (all participants)

Alternative systems of health care including *Yogic method* and psychotherapeutic methods should be adopted more and more.

(Bhattacharjee, Drs. Nizami & Kanti)

More government support, mainly legal and financial, to the NGOs in care of the helpless people is needed. (Punnoose & Kanti)

Mainstream schools and special schools should both be open to each other for integration. (Punnoose, Drs. Nizami & Kanti)

Adoption of very sick children or those having serious diseases involving much money and care needs to be taken up seriously. (Punnooses)

More stringent legal checks on malpractice NGOs in health care. (all participants)

The budgetary allocations in public health care should increase substantially. (all participants)

Mass campaigns for eradicating social taboos and prejudices about diseases, contagious diseases and basic scientific propagandas for social awareness about health, hygiene and diseases. (Mukherjee & Drs. Nizami)

Ethic of public health care be introduced in the MBBS and Nursing training curriculum. (Mukherjee)

Cooperation of the government and private houses in mass health care. (Drs. Nizami & Kanti)

Less segregation in educating as well as curing mentally retarded children. (Drs. Nizami & Kanti)

Involving public in psychotherapeutic method and checks on religious quacks. (Drs. Nizami & Kanti)

Judicious and artful revelation of truth to patients suffering from fatal diseases as well as use of placebos when necessary. (Bhattacharjee, Drs. Nizami & Kanti)

School education should include values of health and hygiene and about diseases and their preventions and cures such as AIDS, Hepatitis B etc. (Kanti).

After all this in the "post-corroboration analysis" we need to reveal the real dynamics of the standard ethical principles and theories though none of our participants (as they accepted) were conscious about applying these things, though strangely many of them spoke of egoism, utilitarianism the *Gitā*, Kant and even theistic ethical theories and empathy. This is possible as I judged owing to their profound study and general awareness along with living in a social life in India having a rich cultural heritage. Much was possible as I still think owing to their being members of a huge ecological community where they gather ethical experience and knowledge. This is revealed further in what was nicely portrayed in the dialogue that is, theory non-cooption in the final consensus and resolution of moral crises in health care. First interesting thing to notice in the entire affair is that though Mariama and the Punnooses based many arguments on the Christian ethic of empathy, which strangely (and truly perhaps) Bhattacharjee accepted as a supporter of *Vedānta* and *Rāmakrishṇa* but was thoroughly rejected by both Kanti (a Hindu by faith) and Nizamis. And yet, in a queer theory non-coopted way or better said in a queer transcendence of ethical or ethical-religious standard theories, all of them accepted that the summum bonum or the ethical goal of public health care ought to be "biological well-being" as mentioned before. Is this a strange affair? Not possibly as none would contest this secular scientific thesis (if I am really allowed to say that), and this theory does not fall under any known or famous ethical theory. Can it be called ethical teleology at best? Perhaps yes, because the inherent sense of "human welfare" which has been further qualified by "biological" amounts to say that higher "teleos" or "purpose" should be there when we are asked about why public health care is morally desirable. Hence, the 'desirability' of the issue of "care" depends largely on a focused "purpose" which is nevertheless, "welfare" or "well-being". However, what we call "welfarism" as distinct from "utilitarianism" (a teleological theory), is much broader than "biological" and "economic" welfarism. Still it makes sense largely within normative ethics which need not be so constricted as not to include them because the said teleological normative thesis is far from being a matter of dispute and so is "welfarism" which, broadly speaking, transcends utilitarian presumption of "maximization of pleasure and happiness" as well as Aristotelian vagueness of "well-being" to spell out good produced over evil in this world in either physical or mental or intellectual or spiritual sense or a cluster of these things, which is good itself or desirable itself and thus desired or to be thus prescribed. Hence, "biological welfarism" is a member of the whole called "welfarism" or one among a concept of cluster of human well-being. Thus from these untrained people in ethics we learn a few things in ethics when we talk to them. Interestingly, not to the least did they give their effort consciously to apply this theory to resolve all critical problems of different nature emerging in health care. Second thing is that the sharp difference in opinion about the ethic of pity, sympathy and empathy amounting to evaluate what virtues count most, they did speak of the value of theistic ethics, utilitarian and even egoistic ethics, but ultimately squared on "sympathy" and "compassion", and as I believe, they did not completely reject "oneness" and "love" but in the midst of all that where did all belligerence about theism, atheism and altruism go? In fact, consensus leaves out several things after moral prodding and in it no one is defeated because all views cannot be ethically admitted by all parties. In a complex multi-lingual, multi-racial, multi-faith nation as India, corroboration of moral views in a democratic way certainly frees itself from the clutches of faiths, taboos and presumptions but equally true is of opinions that finally take a shape. It is exactly due to this that ultimately the thesis of "love" and "empathy" could not be fully trashed as utilitarianism, and even egoism (non-hedonic) found a place. A careful reading of the corroborated points and the rules finalized shows that even the thesis that "selfless performance of duty" without much hankering for what the professional would derive out of it found a place. In fact, intersubjective corroboration is a method that shows us how ethical matters are resolved by constant ethical prodding while transverse views ultimately transcend all conflicts to integrate and converge. The transcendence of ethical theories and principles and yet finding their active presence felt is possible as we find now, it is not mere thinking. Finally, we should say that making a list of virtues and values for humans who happens to be professionals should not be constructed as if the list would enable us to artificially assume such noble characters as doctors or nurses. Virtuous people are not made, they become one in practice nevertheless without consciously knowing that what I am doing now is done by a beneficent person or an honest person or a truthful person. The touted principles in ethics as mentioned here and many more are never adopted as tools by common men, well-read doctors and nurses to resolve their professional crises. Such crises are resolved when they go for moral debates and healthy consensus with an open mind, not prejudiced by theories, virtues, values and principles though they are surely virtuous, they are valuable people so to say even if they were not trained in any artificial way to become one such person. So what do we find? We find that ethical crises in health care, a number of them which we were dealing now or which we came to know in the introduction, are successfully resolved by theory non-coopted people though after they have done such things many theses about ethics come to the fore or some theses emerged of which we had no prior idea. Theories are not intuitive constructions purely; they too come from our experiences in moral life. Theories are also dynamic in dialogues, we need to "discover" as we did here. Readers may now find out many answers to the dilemmas pôsed in the introduction but were not answered in one or the other way. For me, and hopefully for readers of this book, "discovering" from debates and resolutions are more challenging lest we do not merely think in isolation but debate in cooperation. I do *not* assume that what these eight elegant people have said finally is that they have resolved all our ethical issues in health care; they did resolve many of them and must have left many because one course of dialogue is not sufficient – it is a *continuous process* which widens and elevates.

NOTES

1. Buchnan, Allen E., "The Right to a Decent Minimum of Health Care" in Beauchamp, Tom and Le Roy Walters, (eds.), *Contemporary Issues In Bioethics*, Wadsworth Publishing Company, Belmont, 1999, p. 374.
2. Engelhardt Jr., T.H., "Rights to health care, social justice, and fairness in health care allocations: Frustrations in the face of finitude" in T.L. Beauchamp & Le Roy Walters, (eds.), *Contemporary Issues In Bioethics*, Wadsworth Publishing Company, Belmont, 1999, p. 380.
3. Emanuel, E.J. and Dubler, N.N., "Pressing the Physician-Patient relationship in the era of managed care" in T.L. Beauchamp & Le Roy Walters, (eds.), *Contemporary Issues In Bioethics*, Wadsworth Publishing Company, Belmont, 1999, p. 388.
4. Chadwick, Ruth, "Is nursing ethics distinct from medical ethics" in Edgar Morscher *et al.* (eds.), *Applied Ethics In A Troubled World*, Kluwer, London, 1998, p. 124.
5. Kushe, Helga, "A nursing ethics of Care? Why caring is not enough?" in Edgar Morscher *et al.* (eds.), *Applied Ethics In A Troubled World*, Kluwer, London, 1998, pp. 127-142.
6. Harris, John, "Should we attempt to eradicate Instability?" in Edgar Morscher et al. (eds.), *Ibid*, p. 108.

4

Ethical Issues in Donation, Banking and Transplantation of Biological Materials

Choosing the ethical issues in public health care as one important issue in this book is owing to its "universality", that is, the issue is of global importance for the mankind for times to come. Noticeably the issue is of the safe keep and welfare of the precious life, which is unarguably, inherently valuable. When it comes to allied universal issue of keeping the life safe and pleasurable, we may imagine many other issues like, "transplanting organs or parts of organs" or "transfer of biological materials" like sperms, cells, tissues, embryos, fetal tissues and so on. Let us come to consider some of these issues here for they are not merely practical problems for physicians and others; rather they are 'value-laden' problems needing resolution. However, we cannot start with their value aspects abruptly for we have to first consider what these issues are at the practical level. In fact, the exposition of practical aspects needs to be considered along with the value or the ethical aspects. Further, the choice of the issues here have been largely guided by their "appeal", that is, they have extremely widespread impact on our national life because in developing nations like India (expected to be a super-power at some epoch), having huge human resources cannot sheer neglect its value however distasteful arguments for its bane is in the air. Basic sense of economics does not allow us to be so distasteful about it if we really understand its value, though nobody needs a phenomenal increase any more, but that is far from neglecting the value of what we have or the value of management of the present resource. Moreover, certain practical problems of the rise of some dreaded diseases at different locales in India and their subsequent management or safe keeping creates unique ethical furore.

Certainly that needs more care and more allocation from the nation creating some rift for discrimination visible within the national health care strategy. No one among us would be surprised if we ask why on earth Bill Gates is here to pour in funds for AIDS. Or, if we ask why budgetary provisions of health care in eastern states or in Jharkhand (my state) is so poor, when we know that these states are poor in many respects? Hence, some selections of issues here are guided by 'universality' as well as local 'appeal'.

The selection of the issues to be considered in this chapter have assumed great degree of "universal status" because facing more and more nation's life threatening health disorders find it just to fight such disorders with great belligerence even opting for organ transplants. Medicines, mainstream and alternative or whatever, they are no more fondly thought to be only wonder-things which would be sufficient for our well-being and pleasure. No doubt, we need to support these things and be supported by them, but for good results we should care for different sound medical methods of transplants because since long time transplantation grew as a crude business of the quacks operating like mechanics to the ultramodern ways of mending vital organs. It is not true that every other modern state goes for transplants every now and then but the practice is prevailing over many not-so-good cures, and expected to spread. When we come to the cases of donation as well as banking of some vital organs, we become clearer about the fact that some donated and banked organs are not for decorating labs but for placing them at their right places when right time comes for the right person, which amounts to "transplant" them. However, more widespread and old is the practice of "transfusion" of blood, which is an important biological material donated, banked and transferred (not transplanted). Hence, "transplants" and "transfusions" are two modern ways of human well-being and happiness other than administering medicines and other supportive surgical practices. When we come to "transplants", an interesting way is to replace a worn-out organ or part of it by another suitable and healthy one but from a *foreign source*, which is a *non-human source*; this is *Xenotransplant* or *Xenografting* as we call it. It is different from the *human to human transfer* of biological organs and transfusion of blood. It is not true to say that Xenotransplant is a global phenomenon but it is gaining momentum, though human to human transfer of biological substances are common enough. When we come to the unique "appeal" of such methods in biomedicine at local levels, for instance, considering Indian context as distinct from the global context, and within India, a place like Ranchi (my city), they have a different importance altogether. For instance, in India it would be always a different situation for various reasons as and when someone goes for a pig heart transplant or donates body after death for research or for medical purpose or goes for selecting appropriate sperms for medically intervened progeny. Equally important is to notice that at local levels, an instance of malpractice in kidney transplant or some politics in eye banks for a cornea transplant would create different situations of turmoil. Yet, we cannot avoid the truth that speaking globally or locally, these issues affect us positively or negatively not because we are great followers of the intricacies of biomedical science but because they raise distinct "ethical" questions. We are often stimulated to ask: Was it right or just to do such things? Should we allow such things when I or my kin or other are involved? It is not surprising in almost all the cases of transplants and transfusions that such queries are natural because even in the case of blood transfusion, the matter of "paid donation", "black marketing and profiteering" as well as "compulsory tests for HIV/AIDS for the donors" raises many interesting ethical questions. Let us come to these now.

Peter Singer reports in his absorbing essay "On comparing the value of human and non-human life"[1] that in 1991 while he was attending to a talk delivered by a paediatrician in Melbourne's Royal Children's Hospital about organ transplantation, he came across a strange experience of the paediatrician. He was responsible in the care of the young patients in the intensive care unit, one was healthy in every way but faced a grim death owing to lethal heart defect needing immediate "heart transplant". The other patient suffered through brain haemorrhage and declared cortically dead though brain stem still in function, and therefore, not deemed to be "legally dead" but "medically sure to face the fate". In any case this child was having no problem in heart, and breathing and blood circulation still going on. The time was meager but the paediatrician thought that if immediately the heart of this cortically dead baby was removed and transplanted to the one having defective heart, one who was sure to die would save the other having some hope for survival. However, legally that couldn't be done though possible and may be ethically desirable as well. Is it really so? Should we go for heart transplant of the deemed to be dead baby to save another baby who is otherwise healthy and had better chance to survive? It is not difficult for us to imagine a situation when a deemed to be dead old person and a young child injured in a severe accident both needing a rare group of blood for transfusion had to satisfy with only one packet available and no donor around, who should be ethically preferable for the packet though the older one may be undergoing treatment for a longer time? Numerous problems in practical life regarding transplants and transfusion might be faced most likely raising ethical dilemmas for us. Singer reminds us that similar problem arose in 1984 when Dr. Leonard Bailey of Linda University Medical Centre in California transplanted a baboon's heart to save baby Fae thus successfully credited for first Xenotransplant and saving the deemed to be dead baby. However, after three weeks the baby died kicking a long debate for the ethicality of Xenotransplant. Yet, Bailey cannot be sued for he worked under a consent which was ethical but people did not stop talking, neither the physicians. Some said that it was unethical on grounds of gross-egoism and unwanted experiment on transferring an alien organ or that of a different species on humans. The other called it ethical for a ray of hope for saving human species could be seen. Singer thought that a missing argument for unethicality is that "a healthy baboon had been killed in order to provide a heart for Baby Fae"[2] eluded us in the midst of all controversy. This is the line he would himself toe, to which we shall come later on.

In the meanwhile we shall unfold more mysteries shrouding organ transplants and the natural ethical questions relating to this before focusing more on Xenotransplant. We should accept the fact that with the burgeoning growth in modern surgical methods, need for organs has increased because the "need" or "demand" was always felt. In any case with scientific access to organs and the probability of satisfying needs, for which perhaps (partially at least), scientific adventures must have preceded, human organs as well as other animal organs were gradually treated as "commodities". It must be easy for an economist to explain why with commoditization, needs should accompany the idea of "cost" and "purchase capacity". Really such good things for us cannot be obtained free. Organ transplants need not be free-lunch affair. The cost of biological commodities apart, the cost of extracting and grafting, a complex affair involving so many inputs must be high enough. Hence, transplants involve a lot of transaction of money. The donation aspect need not be free either though once in a blue moon if a donor (most likely father or mother of a child) donates an organ free of cost, it is still not "free" because the price tag on the whole biological process extracts money from the free receiver. Or else, if the free altruist donor is unrelated person, does not in any case accept any reward in cash, the recipient has to still afford some good amount to pay for the total process and recovery. And we know well that it is at the cost of the recipient whose purse becomes fat and why. Why at all? Because the person responsible is not an amateur researcher on such subjects, someone who has enough money to be an altruist, rather needs money for the process to continue further and he continues to live perhaps a decent life. So we have at hand some money affair in transplants (and also in transfusion as I believe). It would not be a good argument to cite an example of a non-profiteering government hospital extending transplants to patients "free of cost" because the operating party is paid by an organization and does not do it free. On the part of the recipient, only a fully subsidized pre and post-operative treatment would be in the real sense "free". When everything done in the spirit of benevolence, it may be called "free" lest that happens somewhere because in any case the public hospitals should arrange for procuring such organs at some cost from somewhere by paying from public fund. In any case, the government hospitals do not generate money, they have it from somewhere, from the budgetary allocations of the government or from the tax payers. Hence, there is nothing "free" in organ transplants, it is an intricate web of expertise, need, cost, money, and profits to some but none to others. Hopefully everything is consented and legal. It is assumed that more involvement of money is where subsidies are ruled out, mostly in the private organizations. Yet, experience tells us that in government hospitals "money-game" does float in air for "need satisfaction" at a "high demand scenario" at low or so-called free costs. There is also game of "power" (muscles as well), and a lot of "politics". Hence, in subsidized benevolence, most of the time apart from the factors mentioned above, "power play" and "politics" do have major role to play. We know that history is a testimony to growth and flourish of unethicality where power, politics, power-politics, money, subsidy, need and fight for life commingle, as it does, in transplants of "comodities" called "human organs" and "biological materials". Is it too strange to "commodify" human or non-human animal organs?

There is always a flip side of the coin. Many people argue that in private or public health care centers where organ transplants and transfusion are common practice with large or small amount of price-tag attached to the whole process, it cannot be abused on the ground that some people have deliberately infused malpractices, bad money and illegal procedures because science itself has not asked people to do a nuisance rather, aims at "biological welfare" of global citizens and for that reason there are some non-conventional or ultramodern ways of surgery for cure and care which for their novelty and unique features are difficult to accept for we are most of the time under typical scepticism towards such untraditional things. When the moot point is human's well-being, why should transplants (even xenografts) be called unethical? Moreover, fault finders have bad habit to hide some important truths that mend their psychopathic attitude. There are many subsidized treatments arranged by the government for very poor people and in stray cases even in private hospitals one good doctor acts a Samaritan, taking some money or rather very small amount not for name or fame or for excellence. Should we call transplants bad names when we have experiences of such benevolence? Transplants are, therefore, not essentially money matters, it is something more and even if money does matter for qualitative health care, it is natural. Nothing comes free; benevolence at the cost of begging is not ethical either. If you ought to pay for basic needs, you should pay for keeping life safe and to live longer in happiness.

Here is at hand a good debate, each party armed with their arguments for ethicality of transplants, transfusions and allied problems in donation and banking. However, Singer's question still remains unanswered. He says: 'What is great in scepticism? What is ethical in the killing non-human life by extracting vital organs for the so-called noble ethical ideal of "biological welfare of human beings"? Is such welfare really possible at the cost of ecological imbalance? Another problem unresolved is, should organs of animals, human and non-human be "commoditized"? What is biologically given to us ought to be protected by us for our welfare to the utmost and not to sell it at any cost. Those who are biologically handicapped or deprived need to live with their problems or try for any alternative ways for existence but they have no right to become a party to buying and selling or killing. Why should not science find other ways to save our lives if it is so welfaristic?

This way we can go on and on unravelling so many questions and finding answers but for now I would like to have at least two major issues of *speciesism* and *commoditization* but a few words about organ transplantation situation in India first. India must be in a deep slumber because only a decade back, in 1994 precisely, "The Organ

Transplantation Act" was passed, which was applicable only in a few states. The main reason behind this may be no-threat perception perhaps in our given socio-cultural conditions regarding transplants and their many ethical problems. Or, may be not much could be done before this period by our scientific fraternity in this field. Or, that there was no urge or need for organs to be transplanted for they were either unavailable or beyond the reach of most of the people here. Hence, there must be something happening around in very late 80s or in early 90s which compelled us to wake up from a deep slumber. Global scientific achievements must be one that pushed us. Availability of technical knowledge, equipments and medicines for pre and post-operative care must be other reasons to wake up. Yet, another reason may be change in social perception about health care, investment related to it and change in the role of insurance companies and banks in health care sector. Other reasons may be many, such as increased number of patients needing transplants and spurt in economic capacity to invest in health care. Still, one thinks that there must be a steady increase in the number of our excellent trained doctors who took the challenge of transplant and transfer of biological materials from one source to another. Whatever it may be, in 1996, we found Dr. Dhani Ram Baruah came up with Xenotransplant for the first time in India. He transplanted pig's heart, lung and kidney on 32 year old Purno Saikia suffering from high pulmonary vascular resistance with left to right shunt. Saikia was helpless in going for costly treatment for his nearly hopeless condition leading Dr. Baruah to conduct a *consented research* on Saikia. The person died on the eighth day and Dr. Baruah was imprisoned for 40 days and got out. He approached the National Human Rights Commission for a damage measure of Rs. 5,220 crore from the Assam government because the 1994 Act was wrongly applied and interpreted in his case (and the Act we believe must be too naïve at its inception) and thus preventing him to do life saving humanitarian research. Dr. Baruah said that the Act is only applicable to a human donor who is living and not dead. Hence, an extraction of organs from non-human animals as well as dying and dead humans were perfectly all right if that amounts to a research leading to save lives of humans. Moreover, Dr. Baruah argued that though his subject consented for the experiment, he did not bother taking consent of the pig, it was not his mistake. Dr. Baruah had a battery of disturbing arguments for the infancy of the Act as he charged the state government to not to refer the case to an appropriate authority in Delhi after 60 days of inaction. It was a political move to stop him running his heart research in backward Kamrup district which was backed up by the then chief minister Hiteshwar Saikia. Calcutta based lab. confirmed that the doctor did a systematic Xenotransplant and the patient did live for some time and the Guwahati court found that the said Act was not at all applicable in the state of Assam. Dr. Baruah charged other fellow doctors for connivance while doctors abroad found this possible, such as Dr. Christian Bernard, Dr. Denton Cooley and Dr. Leonard Bailey. Interestingly, Dr. Baruah was said to have operated on Saikia twice, on 15 December, 1996, when he transplanted heart and on 31 December, 1996, along with Dr. Jonathan Ho of Hong Kong and four other attending physicians he transplanted lungs and transfused porcine blood into Saikia. After six years from this event in January 2002, it was reported that in another part of the world female pig cloning was possible (five of them, Noel, Angel, Star, Joy and Mary) which the researchers said would "pave way to transplanting pig organs into people without causing immune rejection". So the objective of the research was somewhat clear. The research was phenomenal as the gene in pig that prompted human rejection (as in Saikia perhaps) was removed thus enabling safe transplant. There was lot of pump in the physicians belly as Dr. David Ayres of the PPL Therapeutics, Scotland who cloned Dolly the sheep said: "Xenotransplantation is the holy grail of the cloning field and the unmet clinical need that can be met here in huge".[3] The project cost was substantial, not affordable by our standards but "they" did it at that cost because at that point of time 75,000 Americans reportedly waited for human organs for transplantation. Readers must be conscious that in the mean time a number of ethical questions that have already emerged made more interesting the cases of Dr. Baruah and Dr. Ayres. We came to know that if Acts are naïve, they do not support our ethical basis of evaluating something as right or wrong. Moreover, researchers like Baruah do have some benevolent motive for humans but do not suffer any emotive or ethical set back when it comes to animals. For them speciesism is ethically justifiable and legal. The case also focuses the problem raised by Saikia's "consent" because subject's consent raises a set of ethical questions further as we cannot rule out coercion, bribe and exploitation. Dr. Baruah must know well that pigs are not easily available for heart extraction. They have to be either purchased or caught or stolen or domesticated, and for that reason though the pig had no human language to "consent",

consent was still necessary from a human community that constitutes either Indian Medical Association, which hopefully has an existence somewhere in his state or the State Government's Health Department if truly the research was humanitarian but not anti-animal. Dr. Baruah is not comparable to a poultry owner or an owner of meat shop who does not need "consent" of animals for selling and killing, though poultry owners as I know are expected to seek permission from responsible authorities before starting business. Dr. Baruah should have remembered that in researches involving animals as *means* and man also as a *means*, some competent authorities need to be approached or else if he smelt there were many loopholes in the Act and still it was important to do his work, why did he not knock the door of justice to enable him to bypass the Act or to modify to suit his case? Because he smelt, if he did, he would be prevented by tight capping the legal loopholes. So was it ethical in any case to act in stealth and cunning involving the one (Saikia) who had speech but was allured for life to keep silent, while the other who did not speak, was killed? Yet, Dr. Baruah's foreign friends might reply: "look, at many places where people do not pop up like popcorns as in India, we have dwindling population, the sick ones threatening it most but plenty of money is available to treat them. So let pigs be sacrificed for humans if needed. Dr. Baruah may not argue this way but he would toe the old line to argue that stealth and cunning are desirable for a "greater good". When social agencies are so foolish as not to respond to health care taker, a sane person has to take charge to save mankind even at the cost of a pig. Much like "Drowning a thousand dogs to save a person on a sinking ship". So the ethical imbroglio continues. Are you disgusted? Not so much as I believe because you feel that "your" answers are not sacrosanct; ethics is a field of disagreement which gives way to agreement if we have applied a method, but for that we shall wait.

Now it is important to come to a more micro-level for another interesting phenomenon in transplantation. This time a human kills another to save yet another, the second one has a fat purse, the first one gets fat by having some from the second, while the third has none, so he dies. Dr. S.S. Prasad a famous nephrologist of Ranchi was charged with illegal organ-trade because he has been involved in a kidney-racket the base of which is Prasad Nursing Home in Ranchi and spreads its tentacles to Mumbai and elsewhere. Dr. Prasad was sent to jail on May 5, 1998. This was perhaps a good follow up report after Dr. Baruah's benevolence. Local newspapers reported that the charges were framed on Dr. Prasad as based on the testimony of a poor Mumbai power loom worker, Nasir, who said that one of his kidneys has been taken out without his consent and knowledge by sheer treason in connivance with Dr. Tabrej and Nurse Mary who brought him from Mumbai to Ranchi for treatment. Later, the booking clerk and nurses at the Nursing Home confirmed Dr. Prasad's illegal practice along with an international gang. He was alleged of eight kidney transplants in last two years in treacherous connivance and malpractice. Most interestingly the recipients were all foreigners and Dr. Prasad was assisted by doctors and surgeons from Mumbai. Under tremendous public pressure the Indian Medical Association of Ranchi Chapter had to accept a few truths but allegedly while police probe was still on, the Chapter resolved that it was "technically impossible" for a transplant patient to be brought from Ranchi to Mumbai in an unconscious state, meaning thereby that the subject was himself under cloud. Yet, under the police probe it was learnt that our doctor said he wanted the Nursing Home to be the saviour of kidney cases in eastern India, especially Bihar (Jharkhand came into existence in 2000), but there was poor flow of kidney patients here causing some problem for monetary recovery of what he had invested. Another interesting photograph was available (subsequently published in *The Times of India*, May 31, 1998) showing five recipients at the Nursing Home, while one among them was an office employee having good health and thus a fake case of transplant. We will not go into what happened further because we have some interesting things for our purpose inherent in this story. Is it ethically permissible for our community to have such free practices of organ transplants, in private nursing homes as serious as kidney transplant without many checks on the practicing people, particularly when these hospitals run by a person or a small group invest much but soon run out of the fund? What is the ethical validity of permitting such Nursing Homes (under the government permission so to say)? Interesting arguments emerge here when we learn that in some government hospitals the in-house doctors who do a more of out-of-the-house job, are first involved in sabotaging the in-house systems of transplants and then outsource the jobs where they do it at good price. There might be a well knit in-house nexus and for that reason a subsidized malpractice might soon flare up even in public hospitality. These are not imaginations, if there are conscious people who are well-informed, our physicians in particular, must be aware of such things. The question is, when this is the situation in the government hospitals, why should we not go for private care? What do we find when the public health caretaker turns cold face? No sooner you ask this question, another one makes it a full circle: Should we then go to the private houses which runs for profit and mostly built and run by fishy people already attached to the public institutions? Another fresh set of questions are needed, like, what would our hundreds of poor kidney recipients do when private houses are unaffordable and mischievous? What if public health care institutions fail? Hence, questions of transplantations take us to interesting realms of politics, economics, power and power-politics. More interesting for me though, it takes us to consider the motives of profiteering, maximization of ego satisfaction, greed, malevolence, treachery, treason, bluffs, exploitation and unethicality permeated all around. It takes us to consider the medical fraternity's ethical status, courage, wisdom and urge to benevolence in this poor country. We question the ethic of a poor guy to be bluffed, made unconscious and his kidney extracted. We question the IMA to issue a consensual decree which is under cloud. We question the poor clerk to be posed as fake recipient and the courageous people of an institution suddenly turning approvers under police probe but not acting *whistle-blowers* before that. Do we need more in-house whistle-blowers in such hospitals? We should answer these questions before we call ourselves a good name—"civil citizens". These questions are not posed by Singer because these are not about favouring one species over another in medical care (speciesism), rather favouring one clan over another, the first has fat purse, the other does not have it. These are about who should purchase what, how and why in the name of medical well-being, much of which is to be seen in the case of "commoditization" of human and non-human organs. We might ask Singer a nice question in this regard: Does the ethic of favouring human clan in health care outwit ethic of speciesism? Is the case of Baruah's Xenotransplant of equal ethical importance to the case of human kidney extraction to transplant it to a poor person through treason? In fact, ethic of transplants needs to be carefully discussed when we consider Xenotransplant involving non-humans for organ trafficking and human to human transplants.

Before coming to this weird realm of ethics of transplants we should notice that everything is not quiet in many other cases of using human donated organs after being painstakingly stored or banked.

Let me first say that in case of kidney, cornea, blood and many other "donations" of crucial human materials there are some interesting ethical questions related to banking as well. Hence, ethical questions do not emerge only in case of transplantations rather when organs are "donated" and "banked". Further, there are interesting ethical questions in the allocation of banked organs when they are in need. Not only this, with the growing trends in human need owing to modern ways of living in different cultures and the welfare perceptions changing rapidly, we no more restrict our ethical discussions about kidneys, blood, cornea etc. rather include discussions about sperms, stem cells and umbilical cells. Before turning to these questions, I would like to consider the case of use of the celebrated cells and sperms. We should not forget that in such cases of using biological materials, the "commoditization" thesis may be treated as extremely important and in such cases, human to human transfers are crucial ruling out charge of speciesism. We should not also forget that in "commoditization" cases, power, politics, power-politics and money play vital roles. Perhaps ethics pervades all these things.

It is a global trend and also prevalent in India that major population goes for tubectomy and not vasectomy when it comes to population control through sterilization methods. In India and China the population problem is grim, and in India, in particular, the preference of vasectomy is almost the same through more than three decades though crores have been spent on advertisements of vasectomy. Vasectomy is disliked due to two reasons: damage of male virility and love of children. The first one is a proven ugly myth nurtured by male chauvinists whereas the latter one is a truth. What if a child or children of a couple dies when the male partner has been irreversibly sterilized though they would prefer their own progeny and not any other compensatory ways? One way must be "sperm banking" because one wonder thing has been made possible, "liquid nitrogen". Hence, we cannot first of all pooh! pooh! the call for having sperms donated and stored or banked for further use. Here, one should notice that when we speak of "donating" sperms it is necessarily not restricted to a preconditioned label like, "this sample awaits use if and only if such and such needs it". However, this belongs to such and such with such and such "biological specifications" may be a valid noting on donated samples. Hence, there would be essentially a "biological probability" and "practical possibility" of using or allocating sperm samples to different recipients though "consent" of "concerned party and/or parties" should be available. This does not rule out, therefore, that though donation itself is not necessarily "conditional", its use may be so. Equally true is that there are chances of more "universal use of sperms" as well but that does not merely depend on consent rather on complex social settings, taboos, education and acceptance. In any case the sperms are available for use even after 25 years if banked with precision and act wonderfully as an element of "safeguard" for the people opting for *irreversible* vasectomy. Interesting feature of this banking with the help of "cryopreservation" is that in the process weaker sperms fade out, thus lowering the chances of birth defects and miscarriages when used at a later stage. This is ethically thought to be justified because apart from other things it enhances the success of sterilization programmes much needed for males in overpopulated nations. It is doubly ethical for it is pro-poor and thus non-clannish as the cost of donation; banking and use are within affordable limit and may be even subsidized without much burden on the exchequer. It is been deemed to be ethical because it raises hope for progeny when dear ones have been lost causing much emotional trauma. It has also been taken as ethical in the vastly changing perception of biological well-being of people across the globe because many people are not too fussy about using donated sperms of another person that is needed to the utmost. The whole process is seen as ethical because in tubectomy women suffers most for further need of reversal or recanalization disturbs the biological well-being of women. So they may be spared in lieu of a more safe male vasectomy with a follow up sperm banking. It is also said to be ethical because one could just plan family after one child and not wait for more. It takes out much curse of forced planning as well. But there are questions. We shall come to these ethical questions but before that take this: 'Gaby Vernoff gave birth to a bonny baby girl in Los Angeles to create history. For the baby became the first to be born using the sperm of a dead man. Gaby got the sperm from her husband Bruce who died in 1995. His sperm was collected 30 hours after his death at the pursuance of family members by Dr. Cappy Rothman, Urologist. This is nevertheless an offence in Britain.' Though sperms were extracted from the dead even before this case, those were planted to a woman only in Gaby's case after almost a year when she decided in favour of the process. The British law prevented this practice in essence because it was a non-consented unethical practice. The husband of Mrs. Vernoff had no written consent left for use of his sperm in this way, and being wife perhaps does not give any legitimate moral claim deemed to be legal as well on her husband's biological material potent of giving life without valid consent. Does a wife have biological rights like this one? Is prevention of such rights unethical? Or, is it the other way round? Does derivation of sperms amounts to some kind of unethical derogation, defecation, disrespect and dishonour to a dead man? Or, does dead save any biological status to be further derogated, defecated, disrespected and dishonoured if any of his biological material is useful enough for mankind on earth? These ethical questions further take us to the ethic of donation of biological material even when a man is not alive. We believe that Mr. Vernoff must have no idea about using his sperm and thus about donation but had he such idea, still would present law prevent him from doing so after he had died? Is donation at will possible when alive? Do we really enjoy complete biological freedom when alive? Or, should there be laws preventing us to do certain things, alive or dead? Is it desirable to enjoy the right to be believed from our present biological conditions (which may be poor or very bad or not liked even if it is good), and thus "donate" it instantly giving some freedom to take life and then make us more useful? The ethical-legal questions constantly come up, some reaching the realm of mercy killing and assisted death. In fact, Mrs. Vernoff has to go for a legal battle on ethical grounds by showing a videotape in which her husband requested for a child and argued that a man who does not foresee his future of premature death, cannot give a written consent. Similar case was fought in Britain by Mrs. Diane Blood to use sperm of her husband in coma, who would not give consent at that state. She was refused permission first but the legal battle allowed her to use sperms in Centre for Reproductive Medicine in Brussels. What it amounts to us apparently is moral overhaul of a legal system itself or a legal system transcending its factual bindings to enter into a realm of ought and desirable. However, questions linger in our minds as many of us still think that the moral questions either do not make a good case or they are not solved beyond doubt by a few minds here and there in our highly belligerent world. Yes, we must admit that ethical questions about transfer of biological materials as well as banking of these things still make good sense. As it stands now, the moot issue is the one of "commoditization" of biological materials and its ethic. As I have said, we shall come to its deeper understanding in a moment after we have taken some more cases of banking and transfer of biological materials when two or more human beings are concerned leaving aside the trifle of speciesism for the time being.

Now let us come to the holy grail of biology, the celebrated "cells" and our urge to immortality (perhaps). In the recent times biomedical science owing to its penetration in the micro-realm of existence has raised hopes for banking of potent life for a long time at a micro-level. The technology is to store cord blood stem cells so that in the future, cures for acute and chronic leukemia, sickle-cell disease, inherited diseases like B-Thalassaemia, Hodgkin's disease, stem cell and plasma cell disorders and Ewing sarcoma can be found so as to prolong the life expectancy of our beloved progeny. This must be particularly good news for countries like Australia and Canada and many others where available human resource is too costly a gift and one cannot afford taking threats to life lightly. It is not that in India and China parents do not love their children but that the technology raises hope for an already meagre population. Greater hope lies in the effective cure of cardiac, diabetic, Parkinson's diseases and multiple sclerosis, spinal and cord injuries and strokes. Our interest in the age of global medical care and growing medical tourism is to provide cheap ways to stem cell restoration or banking. In India Reliance Life Sciences provides such banking and assured use for these materials at Rs. 27,000 to Rs. 60,000 depending on the period of banking, which is not believed to be whopping at all by international standards. Well, that may be true and sounds good too but there are questions. Take the ethical aspect of "Clannish favours" (if not speciesism) first. Do we think that average Indians as they are now placed here should be allured for a biotechnological investment at the given cost? Is it a public phenomenon or merely clannish? The houses offering these things are certainly "profit making" than non-profiteering and the government hospitals show little or no interest in such matters in a wide scale. Why should the government be so inert at such things? Is it not desirable on their part to give a helping hand at affordable rate if the touted "science reaching the poorest of the poor" is good in fact? Further, who should consent to the process? The mother, who may not be always in a position to consent and the father who perhaps has no moral authority in the matter or may be not alive? Or, is it the other way round? The mother already in the pangs of child birth should be replaced by child's father for consent? Or, still interesting may be the option of an unconsented legalized cutting and storing of cord after birth. In case of an uneducated person or those having little biological wisdom, what should be the role of the physicians or the health caretaker in this matter? What if someone doesn't like the idea at all on grounds of unnecessary intervention in private affairs? We should not shy away from such questions. The moot question again is the "commoditization" of life or stuff potent of life along with finely manipulated ideas of "insurance of life at birth" and "a veiled threat for decay and death" when life has been initiated but not lived any further. Is stem cell banking based on an emotional blackmail and thus unethical?

Let us now come to another interesting case of "banking" of biological materials. Readers should notice that in case of banking of kidneys or heart or sperm or eye or blood, whatever biological material we need for transplants and transfusion for cure and to save life goes under the concept of "donation". Because the materials needed for a shorter or longer safe-keep should come from a source – a biological resources so to say. If the source is human (let us skip pigs and monkeys for the time being), we expect that such "donors" by virtue of wisdom or benevolence or good name or whatever "voluntarily donates" biological materials owned by them at one point in lifetime, which however are extracted either when they are alive or when they are not alive. There is perhaps no known civil nation in present world where law permits extraction and banking of biological materials without "donor's consent" or without "voluntary legally justifiable donation", the reasons being civil nations care for freedom of will, rational choice in altruism and benevolence and a clear distinction among homicide, suicide and natural death. The moment we care for such things in donation and subsequent banking for use of materials in need, we are further faced with the tough questions about the human civil nature, and about allowing forced and unconsented extraction, banking and use of human organs for humans. Tougher questions are about civil human nature to extract and allow non-human animals' biological material for human use, which we have seen, takes us to "speciesism". This is believed to be unethical in some ways because rationality, free will, altruism, benevolence, every so-called human greatness are at stake. In another way we can say that "donation" of biological materials either voluntarily or coercively or by deceit is faced with different proportions in case of humans and in case of non-humans, though in any case, common point is the ethical validity of the "commoditization" of these materials in cure and well-being. Hence, the crucial aspects of the "commoditization" and "speciesism" in the ethic of organ donation, banking and use are unavoidable, whether we consider humans or non-humans at par or differently. I have also hinted before that the ethic of donation is also intricately related to politics, power and power-politics in our "civil societies" lest we realize apart from many irrationalities, the elements of "coercion", "deceit" and "bungling". Let me now add another element—"poverty", particularly in the context of donating, banking and transfusion of blood.

When poor people of poor or rich countries come to realize that many people need them as "donors" of organs or biological materials, more than their rationality and benevolence, what acts as catalyst is "money" *in lieu of* "organs". It is not that affluent people for more affluence do not have the urge for more "money" in lieu of organs. I cannot be boastful of finding not a single case like this one but for the poor, the urge is perhaps more prominent. I am also not boasting about not finding a case of someone not earning a penny out of a bargain of organs even though the person is extremely poor. What I am sure is that in countries in India and elsewhere, a large number of poor people depending on the "voluntary" bargain of organs are a prominent affair. Interesting is to notice that the bargain is "voluntary", and we have mentioned above that normally "voluntary" donations, even if in the fashion of a "bargain" are not uncommon, though whether such things are ethical-legally justifiable is another point, which needs some care in this regard. Further, I use the term "bargain" because the persons concerned in buying and selling have no doubt about "commodity value" of human body and in the "biological market" (which is growing in the global open markets), for every purchase, maximization of profit at even a great loss of life is quite acceptable. It would be interesting to ask whether or not it will be ethical to open a huge human resource market that India has if and only if humans here are bundle of saleable organs that need money for transfer? If globalization is a little too much in this regard (I don't believe so), at least the idea should work in the national market perhaps? The question is can we become good donors at will for money? If we can, is it ethically and legally justifiable? Take legal aspect first. In India, it is an open trade to sell and buy blood and kidneys for instance. There is no hide and seek in this matter, and for rare blood groups or for an extremely urgent need of money, selling kidney is not a hidden matter any more. If such things are voluntary, are they legal as well? What is good in certain things done being illegal though ethically justifiable? There is an apparent tension here between ethicality and legality. The perception of the poor and the needy in such matters is that a friend in need is a friend indeed, the so-called true friend in need is not bereft of any altruistic value. If this be the case, everything done must be ethical and legal. Are things so simplistic? Can we allow a poor selling kidney or blood (taking that the donated samples matches for biological transfer) at some cost without an external intervention? Moreover, can donor choose a receiver? Or an external agency has to do a stringent banking and follow up transfer rules for the receivers on the basis of urgency and/or on first come first served basis? Is it ethically justifiable that I have no say on selection of receivers when I am the most important donor of blood (or even kidney)?

Other interesting questions crop up in blood donation and blood banking which is understood to be holy gift to mankind. It is not uncommon that some private agencies provide good infrastructure for blood donation and banking. After the Supreme Court intervention in "compulsory screening" of all supplies of human blood, some of these agencies are careful enough to go through compulsory tests of HIV, Hepatitis B and other dreaded health hazards before collecting samples of blood though free of cost. The idea of a paid donation is then replaced by "voluntary benevolent donation" without any precondition of receivers' choice. Yet, it is not uncommon that people donate blood in these agencies on the one hand and on the other hand a receiver who happens to be close to donor gets it after a perfect match. Is this ethically justifiable? How should we control the private agencies in these regards? Take it a little farther to make the case more debating. Some private agencies take money (a good amount) after handing over donated blood (free of cost) to the receiver even if they happen to be close to or related to the donor because they are in no case non-profit making organizations. In any case then, "money" comes to limelight, if not for the donor but for the receiver. More interesting is that these houses sell rare group blood at higher prices in need on the ground that such samples often come from "paid donations" or better said, they come from "blood merchants". It is wrong to call only the donors, "blood merchants" because the seller is a party to it. Ethical as well as legal questions creep in here. We need to ask, why should such agencies that buy and sell blood be at liberty in civil societies? Equally important is to ask, if something like blood is vital for life, what is unethical in paying for it? More disturbing questions are: if the government and some non-government non-profiteering agencies run out of wits owing to lack of fund and infrastructure, what is unethical for private houses to go for a blood bargain? And, if the nation is so inadequate to maintain the minimum welfare of a person, then the common man does enjoy right to dignified way of earning money by selling own biological materials. Why should any agency on earth, who failed to look after his welfare, stop him for paid donation provided the professional donor's blood fits the biological criteria for transfusion? Why should great altruists and people for benevolence cry loud against the egoists fighting for livelihood and for that matter they are tested thoroughly before blood donation? When a paid donor's or a professional donor's act of earning for existence is not at par with smuggling, theft, cheating and deceit, why should he not earn because who else than he or she have complete biological right over organs and biological materials? Interestingly, why should a blood donor (or any other donor) be always a "good Samaritan" and not otherwise? Is it proper to argue that human body is God's gifts, and therefore, not to be sold but gifted as Samaritans do? God certainly does not help much in this regard as He Himself is under scrutiny – did He give us this body? Even if He did, He did not give me food to eat and money to exist, so I am at will to sell, where is unethicality then? So a simple theistic way does not help us to come out of these trifling questions in donation, banking and use of biological materials.

Questions do not stop here as donations of biological materials are not restricted to kidneys, eyes and blood; we donate many more organs with greater knowledge of transplants in the field of medicine. It appears that we may donate the entire "body" when we are "dead" for *therapeutic* and other purposes. It is not uncommon to donate our body in totality for its several uses without any payment and preconditions about the exact ways in which it has to be used. However, "dead bodies" do not enjoy same status, that is, a dead body suspected for unnatural death is not at par with a dead body unsuspected for unnatural death. Hence, we have in India clear legal codes formulated mainly for the unnatural dead bodies (Code of Criminal Procedure, 1978 and Coroners Act, 1981). The negative implication of the Act and the Code is that it prevents removal of any organ from the dead body for therapeutic purposes thus stopping all questions about donation and transplants. Tragically there were few emphatic views about allowing removal of donated organs from dead bodies during the early 80s in India, which in one way encouraged trafficking, malpractices and bungling as well. Hence, "positive" ethical-legal views on using organs of dead bodies were needed urgently. However, problems grew worse with the non-availability of a proper definition of "dead", particularly in view of "brain death". The problem is, when do we call someone "dead" beyond doubt so that organs needed for transfer ought to be extracted before the period of anoxia due to cessation of circulation is at minimum. Many people in the Indian medical fraternity in particular are relieved after the Organ Transplantation Act recognizing the legal aspect of "brain death" provided such death is certified by a physician or physicians at the venue of occurrence of death in association with a neurologist or a neurosurgeon. It is believed to be ethically and legally viable to enable doctors to take off life sustaining aids for speedy recovery of cadaver organs with consent. This lessens the agony of attendants, who die a slow death owing to tension and lack of money. This also stops trafficking of organs owing to their paucity. It has been observed that the confirmation of brain death should enable the *genetically related* occupants of the "body" to allow (consent) to extract vital organs but there should be no prevention from any genetically related person in such cases. The wish of the person holding right on his or her biological body must be respected as well. It has been also observed that competent authorities in a prison and a hospital are custodians of those dead bodies unclaimed beyond forty-eight hours, and thus have right to remove organs, but the body is of no use after such a long duration and the brain dead condition would suffice the custodians to act accordingly when a person is attended by no kin or close attendants. In case of live donation of organs, any removal before death shall accompany a valid case of transfer to a near relative of the donor. However, if the donor wishes, his organs could be given to an unrelated person with an approval of a competent committee constituted under the central and the state government vigil, which is so needed for a check on commerce of human organs. A covenant would be thus necessary between the donor and the unrelated receiver in written form ratified by the empowered committee or else, legal transplant will not be possible. The hospitals and physicians are thus relieved of fixing the relations in transfer of materials. In case of live donations to relatives or unrelated persons, therefore, only registered hospitals under the above Act will be allowed to remove, store and transplant organs. Everything said and done, we must remember that the Act is subject to state approval and in India only few states approve it. Hence, the universality of the Act is still awaited and so is the practical benefit of the Act. The death of organs continues with trafficking related to it. There are problems even when the Act is accepted in totality, because fresh set of problems emerge, which are mainly ethical. Greatest problem is about the "selection of kin" in organ donation. Why should such selection be beyond control and vigil when that may be either under pressure or coercion or bribe or unwanted grudge? One cannot rule out "weighing" the cases of need. Take the case of two persons waiting anxiously for kidney to be transplanted on them for bare survival. In case of a live donor, if biological matching overrules any favour for genetic relation, why should "another person" not receive it if he or she has registered first in a hospital or elsewhere where the kin came next? What is more ethical in selecting relatives (genetic) when biological matching allows selection of unrelated persons? Does the donor have ethical right to rule selection because his act being so great, he enjoys supremacy? Is it ethical on the part of a donor to be a chauvinist in party selection? Does he not by virtue of his selection destroy value of benevolence? Compare this donor with a live donor in a hospital who has no one in this world to prefer, a beggar on the street, who has no party. If the live donor does not have preferences in gifting his kidney to anyone needing it first, should he be revered most for his ethical act? Or, compare the brain dead unclaimed body whose vital parts have been extracted by the competent custodians to transfer it to *any other* person in need on the basis of *first come first served* or on the basis of *medical urgency*, should the donor be ethically more benevolent though he would not be hailed for that act? Hence, the question of ethical commendation of donation always stands a good ground for scrutiny. One wonders, whether commendation is at all ethically justifiable in donations of organs? Is it ethically proper for our live donors to satisfy their urge for immortality or their urge for self-satisfaction, name and fame or their urge to satisfy some emotive whims by selecting kin? Equally questionable is to select any person for donation for any motive which is closer to "self" in reality than biological well-being of mankind. We shall soon come to see, therefore, that "donation" apart from speciesism and commoditization is questioned ethically for selection of receivers and for the intricate policies that is easy to detect.

Having all regard for stray cases of *universal nature* of blood donation and its use, let us look at the case of a death in July 1998 in National Health Service Hospital in Sheffield in England. The deceased did not have any wish for transferring his kidneys, though on pursuance, the close relatives agreed to donate them to the hospital authority for an urgent use but the members of the family were *racists* and demanded a selection of receiver who happens to be a white and not coloured person. It is stunning that the British Human Tissues Act (1961) authorizes consented removal of organs by physicians from corpses for welfare of man but is not legally and morally bound to selection of receivers in consultation with the members of the deceased person. In fact, the British Act does not bind the doctors even to be guided by the wish of the donor regarding selection of kin, though a majority of them have reported that Catholics, Protestants and Muslims request for "religious selections" of donated organs. More grave situations would be influencing selection by politicians. Clearly, ethical questions of selection of recipients on the basis of colour, race, sex and religion are good enough to consider. Here also the hidden chauvinism on the part of the donor and his family regarding selection cannot be ruled out because one cannot overlook the fact that after all it is me, who has this body and I give to others. Yet, most interesting reaction came from the then Secretary of the State for Health in these words: "Donated organs are a national resource which is available to people regardless of race, religions, age and other circumstances". The italicized words are of great interest. Is it ethically as well as legally viable to consider donated biological materials (not inert materials) be treated "*national resources*"? Why should any part of my body, donated by me, be treated a national resource? What is the guarantee that the resource will not be used injudiciously in my absence by so-called competent authorities under pressure and politics? Why should I not be a party to selection of recipient when I am alive or when dead, my representative be not a party to stop malpractice? Moreover, as it was learnt later on, the recipient was a white person most likely again on not so fictitious biological ground perhaps, that is, tissue compatibility makes it unlikely that organ from one race be successfully transplanted to another race, sex, and even age. These factors may be considerable for further biological investigation into the practicability of transplantations giving some fillip at least to the ethic of "selection". With this, we have at hand a number of disturbing ethical questions before us about organ donation, banking and transplantations, which are not good to leave out.

As we stand now, Xenografting and other issues in the transfer of biological materials through donation and banking pose several ethical questions, crucial being the scrutiny of the ethic of speciesism and commoditization in donation and transplants. Let us throw some light on what these ethical issues are like. In a seminal piece Peter Singer (1990) writes: "In the traditional Western view, the welfare of non-human animals deserves probation *only* when greater concern for their interest poses no threat to what we perceive as *our* interests"[4]. His stress on "only" and "our" reminds us about the relative importance of humans over non-human animals when it comes to their respective "interests". It would be unwise here to equate the general Indian perception regarding this matter because most of us love camouflaged speciesism than not, though when it comes to intellectual honesty, whatever *Vedānta* and theistic or non-theistic allies amounts to regarding this matter, we do prefer humans over non-human animals when it comes to "interests". One point of preference may be biological evolutionary supremacy, the other ethical-spiritual supremacy, another one, rational supremacy, and above all, our care for animals when perceivably animals have none for us. Hence, the moot issue is if we do not exist, is there no one to cry over the animals? It is due to this that in cases of conflict between humans and non-human interests, we ought to seek for our interests, it is ethically good so to say. This is the simplest way of presenting the ethicality of preferring "our" species and not another species or what amounts to the ethic of "speciesism". However, Singer and his many Indian proponents argue that "we ought to extend the basic moral idea of equality which we apply to all human beings – to animals as well"[5]. These people clarify the sense of "equality" in different terms. They mean to say that humans and non-human animals have "equal consideration of interests"[6] as in cases of "pleasure" and "pain". So it would be a kind of prejudice to champion the cause of human interests only because it is the same as unethical preference of a race or a caste or a class.

With this background to speciesism, Peter Singer comes to the case of Xenotransplant and its ethical aspects because for him this is an ideal example of "speciesism", which is evidently unethical on the simple ground he has mentioned. To be clearer Singer argues that it would have been more commendable for biologists and physicians to conduct transplantations of human heart on another human who needed it most rather than killing a baboon or a pig for getting heart. Or, else there should be no such attempt as we suppose. Let us take death sportingly if that comes to us in the form of a failing heart or kidney, as I suppose. The problem is that if baboons and pigs have their valuable biological life not by virtue of human expertise, humans have no moral right whatsoever to rear them in cages and kill them when they are needed for human purpose, though we deem it illegal to consciously cage and take life of another human (may be one at a vegetative condition) to use his or her organs for the benefit of another person. Singer rightly imagines that the special status of human as prevalent among us is owing to our perception of non-human animals – we take them to be "things for use" or simply "commodities". At one place Singer holds that there is however a distinction between humans and lettuces; it is valid enough to use "things" like lettuces because these things lack emotions, pleasures and pain as we do, and therefore, "equal consideration for interests" does not hold good here. Singer had to make some case of the use of lettuces at least though we all know that the oxygen and carbon dioxide cycles on which life depends, needs humans, non-human animals, lettuces and other small and big plants and trees. We know that life depends on several other non-living things as well. Hence, Singer's argument to use lettuces and rocks (perhaps), but not non-human animals, leaves some gaps for us. This is one important ethical aspect on which we should reflect when it comes to speciesism about Xenotransplant. In fact, the world is full of so many "decent things" (of Singer) and these "things" as we happily differentiate in our perception of the nature, do not necessarily amount to commoditization and insult of other forms of life, say some thinkers opposed to people like Singer. They would say that we do need things for us; even animals are needed, for our existence and well-being, as the animals too need us or perhaps they use us for their well-being. There is no unethicality here – it is but "natural". However, ethicality enters when we start transgressing the judicious limits of using animals and plants for our interests overlooking their interests completely. What this "judiciousness" amounts to is a matter of ecological wisdom, which great amount of study of ecological science necessarily does not guarantee. Hence, Singer's view should have a half-truth only if he accepts "judicious use" of animals. Further question is whether or not Xenotransplant falls in the category of "judicious use of animals" for the benefit of humans, when "benefit" does not amount to what may be called "cosmetic benefit" (if I am allowed to use that term), rather than "life saving benefit". The problem is whether or not "life saving benefit" may be extended to humans at the cost of non-human animal life. Singer asks if saving life is so important for us, why we should not use a cortically dead infant immediately to save another person who has still a future rather than killing a baboon. He emphasizes that in most of the cases many attendants of vegetative people prefer such way of cure. The point, however, is that there is a lot of human intervention in such matters which baboon-clan does not pose for us. Singer argues that any defense of speciesism on the ground that like family preferences we should have species preferences is fallacious because human family preference and species preference are categorically different. The former amounts to what is normal to us in human society, whereas the latter is not so because preferring our species on fictitious grounds are often debated and opposed by members of our species; there is no universal agreement on this matter. It is, therefore, challenged as racists are challenged on their unethical bias. Hence, family preference is not biased as racial bias or species bias. However, a question still lingers in our mind – what would Singer and others do when Katrina hits helpless people and equally helpless animals around us? Whom do we naturally care for or who should be cared first, my children, my family or my neighbours' children or my pets or my neighbours' pets or the zoological park or the sanctuary close to my home? Are people running for their life but not animal life, unethical people? Moreover, if hopes are raised owing to animal cloning resulting into their multiplication, would one animal life be not sacrificed for saving thousands of human life? What if one dog dies for saving five men on a sinking boat? People like Singer would be unfazed at these questions for they are more in favour of anti-speciesism. They would first of all (as has been already hinted), prefer no artificial experiments on animals amounting to their multiplication for human use for that is an unethical project having sole value for some humans. The multiplication might not stop, rather start ruthless use of animals by human beings. More important is to deliberately forget the truth that though a normal baboon killed for Xenotransplant is biologically more valuable than a cortically dead infant whose organ might be taken out with consent, the latter practice in civil societies would be disfavoured because human life even in a vegetative state is thought to be valuable. Or, some believe if we tend to differentiate cortically dead as useless in comparison to another normal person *within* our race, we end up in "Nazism", for it would be ethically just ultimately to exterminate all non-Aryans for the sake of the Aryan race. Hence, taking "right to life" as an ethically sacrosanct idea in our societies, Singer holds that in any case the idea that a cortically dead does not stand as good "commodity" for transfer of biological materials as baboons are is not acceptable to him because the imaginary theoretical threat of Nazism does not prevent him from saying that taking life of humans when they are cortically dead for saving life of a perfectly well baboon would be ethically just. Singer does open a can of worms because apart from many other things, it would be extremely interesting to find out what he thinks next when biotechnological revolution enables human cloning as easy as having hot cakes in numbers and then use one at the very nascent stage for a transplant but baboons would live a happy life in wilderness—unharmed, not cloned. But status of cloned humans as biological commodities for use is another matter though not altogether alien from our discussion of transfer of biological materials.

Much attention has been paid till now on cortically dead humans *vis-à-vis* baboons; we now need to focus more on some ethical aspects of Xenotransplant in particular, thus leaving out human to human transplants. Jonathan Hughes in "Xenografting: Ethical Issues" (1998) writes: "The main consideration prompting current interests (in Xenotransplant) is the shortage of donated human organs. Xenotransplantation, it is hoped, will close the gap between the number of patients in need of transplanted organs and the number of organs available. The moral importance of treating more patients and of funding better treatments should be uncontroversial.... The ethical problems raised by Xenotransplantation will... be considered under the following headings: (i) interfering with nature, (ii) effects on the recipients, (iii) effects on other humans, and (iv) effects on donors"[7]. It is interesting to notice that Hughes sidesteps any hackneyed way of analysing the ethic of Xenotransplant on the basis of maximization of good of patients. This is but natural that Xenotransplant is in essence a favour for the sick human race that is under pressure owing to paucity of vital organs which are so needed to do the favour. Taking this for granted, we should better scrutinize the ethic of Xenotransplant from other angles. Naturally one way (as Hughes mentions) is to find out whether or not it is ethical to interfere with the basic ways in which nature and natural beings exist and whether or not undesirable effects could be seen on the donors and the recipients. If one can successfully show that Xenotransplant does undesirably affect the nature, natural beings, the donor and the recipients, it is in essence ethically bad and not good. Hence, the practice may be shunned in our society. Let us consider these points as these will give us a cue to what charges of unethicality is often labelled against Xenotransplant and the way in which they may be refused, and this is a good ground for our readers to sharpen their minds regarding this matter when they come to know in the last part of this chapter a real life debate about Xenotransplant and consensus emerged after intersubjective corroboration. One argument against ethical validity of Xenotransplant is that doing so some biologists interfere with some beings in nature or, so to say, nature itself in part at least, which is essentially *unnatural*, that is, "not expected on the part of human nature" to do such things. Hence, certain human actions are "according to their basic nature" or to use Aristotle here, certain things we do *qua man*, which is natural and others quite unlike us are "unnatural". It amounts to say, therefore, that any unnatural human act is not good in itself rather, ethically undesirable or bad in itself. Xenografting being one such act is ethically undesirable. We are aware with an extreme vision of this as: 'God has given us human nature and we are expected to act accordingly or else, we are unethical'. The counter argument is equally emphatic. It holds that God or no God, humans *qua* humans have "nature" unique to them, and apart from much such uniqueness, one is to interfere and manipulate with natural beings and things which makes humans the most evolved race perhaps. Naturally, therefore, humans should (ethically) interfere with nature, that is, it should take out organs from non-human animals if needed for their race to be good enough to exist. Hence, man *qua* man should by nature Xenotransplant and thereby be ethically good. Moreover, if certain biological (medical inclusive) acts of trained humans are natural and some are unnatural, how do we make such distinction? Do we say that at one time when medical quacks gave no medicines to a person down with chicken pox was "natural" whereas those who prescribe medicines antibiotics act unnaturally? I feel amused to say that in India, even today, among some educated people, chicken pox is a boon on man by benevolent goddess and one has no ethical right to intervene by inoculating and/or medicating. Interestingly, these people, unknowingly perhaps, *treat* these infected people with margosa leaf, its oil and turmeric as and when needed. Now, for us, *In Vitro* tests and Xenotransplants have become "unnatural" but why is it so, is not known to us? On fictitious grounds of "naturalness", Xenotransplant cannot be deemed "unnatural" and thus unethical. Why should unnatural acts of man be unethical? Logically speaking, unnaturalness is not necessary and sufficient ground for unethicality. In fact, human beings since time eternity have been doing many unnatural things which are not unethical. They have interfered with nature's fury, diseases, famines, floods with unnatural vengeance, which is not unethical. Apart from so many biological-medical marvels man has invented many things by challenging natural courses, which are boon and not bane, and for that reason, not unethical. Hence, if through transplant of pig heart with supportive care for immunosuppression, man is able to save precious human life on earth, it is ethical though unnatural in the sense of an apparent "incompatibility" between animal organ and human organ. Yet, belligerent people argue that certain natural facts, much beyond our control and manipulations which are crucial in understanding what is unnatural and thus unethical for us to do. We cannot just stop death by any biomedical ways but we strive for it, which is an unnatural act, and to run foolishly after it, spending time, energy and money, everything should be unethical therefore. It appears that Xenotransplant is one foolish way to immortalize the biologically mortal man, it should be thus, unnatural and unethical. Still Hughes and many others argue that Xenotransplant is not human interference with natural fact called "death" and this to immortalize man, rather to find one way to prolong good life on earth which is often cut short by a failing organ. As death is natural to us, that we realize, but for the physicians it is essentially immoral to allow death by no intervention rather, to fight with all might so that human life, precious on earth is lived in the way it should be. We may argue that Xenografting is one important humane way to overcome the given "natural structure" of our "biological organism" but not to change it in any sense. It is also to accept the limitation, that we cannot immortalize man by Xenografts. Hence, physicians and researchers have ethical ways of looking at the biological organism. In fact, the fear of the success of Xenotransplant in the face of the structured limitations of man is an unfounded one, which is prevalent among theists believing in God's Creative Act, an Act which is sacrosanct. The "fear" really is about a likelihood of decreasing faith in Creator God, but may not be loss of faith in God Himself.

Even if we do not overplay with the idea that biological organisms are God-gifted, says the opponents of Xenotransplant, we have to accept the truth that the practice does blur the difference between non-human animals and humans, which amount to an emotive shock for the recipient as well as for a large number of his or her associates who would find apathy for a "man with a pig's heart" because for them the body is maligned by a "lower being" so nasty and hated for its way of life. Hence, by maligning human nature and giving it an indefinable status in animal kingdom, we do great disservice to the person in particular and humanity at large, which is, therefore, unethical. The supporters of Xenotransplant laugh at such ignorance because lack of biological wisdom amounts to say all this. It is possible only in mysteries and fictions that having an evil heart, one goes evil. Truth is that pig's heart might beat exactly as ours do and the biologically fit person who was erstwhile degraded to a useless vegetable suddenly spurts in human activities (not like pigs, any way). Hence, as pig's heart does not turn us to pigs but revitalized humans, it is ethically justifiable.

Coming now to the next point, that is, effects on the recipient Hughes reminds us that we cannot reject the possibility of "rejection of transplanted organs" and "infection resulting from immunosuppression" in cases of Xenotransplants. However, such risks are there in human to human transplants of organs as well. Anyway, we cannot overlook the factors of effects on recipients in Xenotransplants. This is doubly true if you believe the antagonists because for them such effects enable us to charge unethicality. The reason being that even if a person "consents" for Xenograft knowing serious risks mentioned above, "consent" itself cannot be the basis of ethical justification of the practice because the *so-called* consent is an emotional decision or a blackmail of a person leaving all options to live but accept this extreme one. The consent being irrational, emotive and hurried calls for a sane practitioner to overrule such requests and not to take "risks" when it is really proved to be very high indeed. This would be thus for the good of the person and others who follow him or her and, thus, ethical. No doubt, a recipient should be well acquainted with the "high" risk factors in Xenograft, there should be no hide and seek or blackmail and that mere hopelessness or mere heroism does not govern Xeno-experiments. Yet, if someone is able to overcome these things, as we come across many such people across the globe since a long time who volunteered for a rational altruistic good for all future beings to infest earth, Xenotransplant should be given a chance, says the protagonists. Only through risky though careful experiments did bio-science give us good life.

The antagonists would still be dissatisfied as they would now draw our attention to "effects on other humans". These people argue that Xenotransplants are clearly risky affair and we cannot overrule the possibility of fatal diseases of unknown types spreading from a recipient to the societies at large causing great harm to mankind. We are these days cautious after bitter experiences with AIDS, SARS and Foot and Mouth diseases. Who knows what more is in the offing when a pig heart transplanted person starts living with people who had nothing to do with betterment. The truth is that apparent short lived good of the recipient would be incorrigible further through infections and be transmitted to uncoopted persons. This is clear injustice on the part of the recipient and the physician and thus unethical. Hence, costly Xenotransplant experiments would be sheer wastage of money and energy for something evil follows from it, and thus, undesirable. More serious is that a recipient might show signs of serious infections after a prolonged incubation period of the same in receiver's body, and thus spreads its deadly tentacles constantly without being clearly and emphatically quantified for the measure of degree of risk of infection and its spread in society. This is to play with fire as if knowingly just for the sake of experiment and benefit of a person and thus unethical. Tragedy is that any fool-proof system is not available to us that can emphasize the risks on recipients now, and if infections of serious kind flare up soon, still worse problem would be to deal with these patients in our society. We are well aware of this problem with the surge of AIDS epidemic. Hence, any bungle with high risks would be inviting greater danger for mankind and thus unethical. Unfazed protagonists are great optimists because they argue that history of biomedicine is a testimony to the fact that great inventions always associated with grueling series of tests on animals and human beings for a near fool-proof success is a tale of loss of some lives and gain of many more. There has always been care for what likely evils would follow, what evil prospects Xenotransplants might have in the future, and the ways in which they may be faced. In fact, we need not stop researches for a greater benefit in the field of mass health care. Hence, fear perceptions themselves are pessimistic, they prevent us from positive action, disengage us from maximization of health care for the public and thus unethical. Moving forward with some risk is thus welcome.

Finally, we come to the ethical problems regarding effects on donor animals because any sane biologist would not dare say that animals are of little concern to them lest they have taken their first lesson seriously. Hence, one has to consider the effects on animals who happen to be donors for a greater human benefit but themselves not likely to benefit from the act. Antagonists' popular arguments include among others, unconsented and arrogant experiments on animals as if they exist in nature to be used in that fashion. This is however grossly against the balance of nature and thus unethical. Further, animals cannot be scapegoats or sacrificial objects for human good because they are not in nature for such things though counter arguments if favour of meat-eating does not hold good in this case because *relation of user and used* in nature in case of meat-eating is not comparable to use animals in Xenograft. Hence, any use of animals as in Xenografting cannot be ethically justified. Further, Xenotransplant might need either cloned animals genetically well-mapped to be free of diseases or they have to be reared with great care safeguarding from all infections. In both cases, *isolation* is needed followed by killing, which is against the basic freedom at natural settings on earth, such isolation is against animal nature and thus unethical. Cloning pigs for Xenograft in good numbers, is equally condemnable as the species is treated merely as objects having value only for experiments and nothing else. The fact of existence of pigs on human mercy is itself unethical. The protagonists have two ways to face this issue. In a relatively softer way they say that our capacities, value, aspirations are much greater than the pigs and, therefore, pigs should be used as donors for our good. The stronger version holds that along with pigs, persons who are brain dead or are in dire vegetative states should be donors (and killed for that matter) provided organs needed are in proper state. In any case, therefore, Xenograft is good itself as a few animals and humans should be used for a greater health cause, and least doubt should be there that it is we who care for animals, either domestic and wild. There is no need to project us as barbaric when despite our concern for good of animals we kill some of them and despite being humans we need to kill some of our race as well who are deemed to be dead for greater good.

With this I would like to stop puzzling our readers any more as a number of trifling questions already haun't us. In fact, reading those does not itself help much, talking about them to find a way out of impasse does help us. However, we have still not in view the ethical jargons in "commoditization" and "donation" in Xenotransplant as well as in human to human transplant. Let us consider them now. Commoditization of *biological materials* range from organs like kidney and cornea to gametes, genes and blood. These "commodities", if we can really use this term, often go along with the idea of "donation" but to classify it, we should better speak of "paid donation". Hence, we can discuss the ethic of commoditization of human biological materials in relation to paid donation of such things. Clearly we have two standpoints regarding this matter. The protagonists uphold the idea that buying and selling of organs as commodities and donating them at some cost are ethically justifiable, the grounds of which are many and not one. The antagonists on the other hand argue that cost, caring and profiteering through marketing these materials in health care market are essentially unethical for reasons more than one. As usual, for our readers, we shall provide a range of debate without much comment on our part for that is not our "methodology". It is not essential for us to refer to commoditization and donation of kidney only, we may now refer to any one of the above organs or vital parts of the human organism. We may now refer to buying, selling and donating reproductive materials and blood, though some hints about these issues have been already given.

The main ethical argument in favour of commoditization and paid donation of biological materials (I prefer this relatively wider notion), is that there is growing scarcity of these materials all over the world owing to several reasons in modern world. Recipients of such materials have increased phenomenally. It is not merely owing to huge population increase but owing to many things, among which most important is access to these materials as provided by the technological advances in their transfer and parallel advances in drugs needed as backup means. Reportedly, Jewish law permits the sale of organs if the removal is not against the well-being of the donor. In VI Congress of the Asian Society of Transplantation in Manila, Father G.W. Healy quoted Pope Pius XII saying: "in case of cadaver corneal donation it is too far to declare immoral every acceptance or demand for payment"[8]. Similarly, the 1977 Bellagio Task Force Report on Transplantation, Bodily Integrity and International Traffic in Organs held stressed there is not a single ethical principle that would justify a complete ban on the sale of human organs under all circumstances. In the celebrated medical journal, *Lancet* (352, 1998) a paper by A.S. Darr and others drew wide attention about the "sale" of kidneys, which was supported by number of writers later on because ethically speaking, it amounted to greater human good and not bad. In fact, people argued that universal ban in its sale are ethically bad. The ethic of sale of life saving human organs is based on the idea of "regulated" but not ruthless sale, which is assumed to increase their supply subsequently saving many lives, which is very tough to neglect by a staunch ban supporter. Another ethical point is that in the process of transplantation hospitals, laboratories, pharmaceutical companies, physicians and surgeons all make financial benefits because neither the operation nor subsequent care and cure come free of cost. It is very difficult to imagine that any agency would give a free lunch at the cost of bankruptcy. Hence, it is ethically justifiable for the organ donor as well as to take some money though by that his or her altruism is not a trifle degraded. One cannot really understand why in organ transplants all is desirable when donors become physically and financially bankrupt. Moreover, one may argue that if not by smallest amount of altruism did someone gift an organ but having interest on personal benefit or personal good by earning money, then why should such egoism be ethically bad when the gift was so good for the recipient? People like Darr argue that when we consider a case of a living kidney donor, they may be of five types: the genetically related, emotionally related, genetically unrelated, rampant profit maker and black-marketer and coercive criminal. Among these, first three are good enough to be called "donors", who may nevertheless ask for some money, which is however, a matter of socio-cultural evaluation for goodness rather than any definite principle based absolute badness. It is exactly due to this that Francis Moore rightly thinks that in Indian socio-cultural perspective selling kidneys from a living donor of the first three types as mentioned above are perfectly ethical whereas two later types are not, that is, the act of paid gifting is neither ethically absolutely good nor bad. Obviously, when money is earned coercively, deceitfully and rampantly, we call it unethical though in the process recipients gain much. Darr thinks that ethical paid donation of transplantable materials need grey-basket economical scrutiny because in that way we consider more ethical ways to donate materials to the needy, the persons who could not afford money, and cry for equality and justice, but in any case that does not amount to pure altruism of a foolish type where donors do not make merry but others do so. However, the wise economists would equally emphasize the possibility of the growth of black money when life's demands meet scarcity and cost. Economists like Gary S. Becker (Nobel laureate) thinks that therefore, introducing market mechanisms will face the scarcity of organ effectively, and in doing so we may consider the possibility of sale and purchase of cadaver organs at a rationally determined procedure. Many protagonists of organ trade and paid organ donation thus believes that the economic wisdom is spreading with banning rampant organ trade and black-marketeering but most importantly encouraging brain stem death criteria, cadaver donation and withdrawing government sanctions in widespread end stage renal diseases. In fact, much antagonism of paid organ donation and organ trade is emotive rather than rational though emotions do not count much in ethics and economics and ethics of economics. The case of organ trade and paid donation being value-laden, it needs adequate ethical scrutiny than emotive outbursts.

Considering the ethical aspect of "commoditization" of many other human biological materials like "reproductive materials" pose different set of problems though we know very well that these materials stand good chance of transfer through trade or paid donation. In fact, something that is "commoditized" is a "property" that in essence can be sold, bought and rented because such properties are *alienable*. However, not everything is an alienable property, rather there are non-alienable properties, not to be "commoditized" therefore, as is with voting right as our property. There is no doubt that even if some properties are commoditized we should put certain checks on their transaction like "ethical checks" because we cannot, for instance, go on buying and selling kidneys at will and by coercion and deceit. However, there are certain commodities the transaction of which needs no such checks such as legally non-litigated plot of land for need of money. Biological materials are thought to be either commodities of free transaction or they are not, but in one restricted sense at least, they are our property to be sold and purchased no doubt. There has been a long hesitation in the history of philosophy to regard some of our biological materials as commodities until the English libertarian philosophy championed by John Locke did not argue forcefully that "my body in the whole" is "my property", I enjoy complete moral right over the "commoditization" of its parts whenever deemed necessary and also practically feasible to do so. As such we hold complete right over any "product" of our body or those we acquire through some personal effort. This has been refined in later times by Robert Nozick[9]. In bioethical literature, writers like L. Andrews (1986), C. Campbell (1992), R. Scott (1981) and M. Swain (1990) substantiate this view.[10] (We have seen that people like Darr are of the same view.) These people argue that "body is a property to be commoditized" is an ethical view because the Principle of Autonomy holds well, that is, the principle by virtue of which our autonomous choices and actions implies our absolute control over body. All body parts and body products that collectively make our "body" are the one which is my property and it is the individual who should voluntarily allow any medical intervention over his or her body for some good. Hence, I allow an intervention of organ extraction or transfer of materials may be for the biological good of another person though personal good is not ruled out when it comes to earn a suitable amount in doing so. It is a debated matter though that the autonomy to allow intervention is primarily for my good or another person's good or both. Unless and until I conceive of my body (in whole) as my property, it cannot be commoditized and thus sold or rented. Now here we must not come up with the glorification of sex perversions or prostitution because that is not a biological gift at some cost for therapeutic purpose rather biological risk behaviour at some gain but great loss. Hence, the popular emotive gimmick that 'commoditization is prostitution' is a wayward comment. Interesting is to notice that "my consent" in medical intervention is also a testimony to "body as my property". Further it is also interesting to notice that this ethical justification mainly holds good in case of "living bodies" and not cadaver or even brain dead persons or those in a critical health state unless there is a will or a wish at least in written or recorded form while one is living a life of active decision-making freely. Controversy may be raised particularly when in the absence of such testimony to gift body willfully at some cost, family members are asked or encouraged for such paid gift or even for free, when clearly the dead or vegetative body is not property of relatives or family members and cannot be sold as per the requirement of the basic principle of autonomy.

Things are not so simple for the protagonists as the conception of "my body is my property and thus to be commoditized" is itself challenged even though the principle of autonomy holds good on the ground that I exist in this biological form and control such existential state does not provide any ethical ground to say that (a) what exists is first of all a property, (b) which belongs only to me, (c) which unrestrictedly should be sold and rented, and (d) which should be restrictedly sold and rented. Moreover, antagonists hold that owing to exploitation, lack of informed consent, risk elements perceived by donors, malady in control mechanism of sale of organs, playing in the hands of the affluent for transaction and the erosion of altruism, the whole affair of paid donation and commoditization is ethically repugnant. Many protagonists have, however, successfully refuted that exploitation, lack of informed consent, risk elements and other issues may be sorted easily when it comes to a careful strategic organ donation system. In fact, much scepticism regarding this matter is due to the wrong conception that a trade in organ must be accompanied by all sorts of wrong ways of profiteering and not by good ways. Even if in trade practices there are lurking dangers, the point is to overcome them and not to be their victims. However, the antagonists are encouraged by an argument provided by Immanuel Kant, the celebrated ethicist. In the *Groundwork of the Metaphysic of Morals*, Kant argued that as human beings as such have some intrinsic value which is unconditional or absolute, they should not be treated as mere means or commodities to achieve an end like profit. Human beings as such are thus not valuable as means rather they are valuable in themselves. Hence, Kant's call is to treat humanity whether one's ownself or any other as "end in them" not as means. Given this maxim, we are not able to justify our perception of human body as property of market value and nothing else. Any intentional act of commoditization and paid donation is thus the violation of human dignity and inherent value. Man *qua* man thus loses its inherent nature or is derogated beyond imagination, which is unethical. To this it may be added that many theists and other spiritualists do not think that a person's body is exclusive to him. Some say that it is the creation of the Divine, others say that in essence it is manifested divinity and many others more realistically hold that the body which exists owing to biological parentage, nurtured and nourished by parents with great pain, cared by the society and nation for growth and development, cannot be an exclusive property of an individual who enjoys the right to sale and purchase. How can human beings be grossly taken as "resources" for earning even if in the process someone is gifted new life? How someone having a shorter in human society who is thoroughly helped by others including natural things and beings be so egoistic and arrogant to sell or lease some of his or her parts for earning? Moreover, if donation is so important, can it be not free from personal benefits? If it too odd to conceive of people who gift an organ on altruistic grounds without any idea of prize, praise and profit? It there is at least one person, who is not profit-making, is he or she a fool or is unethical? Is it not true that we are members of "kingdom of ends" and not means and thus need not commodify any of our, or another person's organs for mere livelihood or benefit or profit? The protagonists however are not satisfied with what Kant says because they show that Kant himself drew distinctions within the nature of a person as having physical body, reason, emotions, feelings and so on, thus allowing us to say that human body may be treated differently by rational people, not as sacrosanct entity but one of great use to humanity. Without any disregard or dignity of such a thing, we should use bodily parts for a greater benefit which is itself good.

The protagonists also argue that the antagonists mostly have a wrong "organic" conception of body and its parts. Even if we allow that myself, the person has this body which is a "whole" consisting of several distinct parts and that without all these parts we cease to exist, we need not think that, therefore, our body (whole) is equal to parts (organs) and that losing any part or some parts would amount to cessation of the whole or myself as a person. My existential personhood is not merely dependent on some parts as existing or not existing at all. Moreover, when we cut hair and nails and pass stool or urine or give blood, we have least notion of losing anything at all – the whole body is not trifle disturbed. Similarly, when we voluntarily give a kidney (not both because that is not needed, no one asks for such things), or any vital part for saving another life and then earn something, we are not bargaining our bodily identity or our personhood or our character. We are in no case maligning what we have or we are not derogating our "possessions". However, the antagonists argue that no fool thinks that when we donate a part we lose our body or we are lost, but it is natural to think that whether or not the way something was given was ethically desirable because in paid donation of a commodity the way was to "earn as much out of transaction" but not "to save life". There is a gap left here however for unpaid, pure altruistic donation at will escaping commoditization, which is often hailed and not hated. Equally true is that a gap is left to ethically curse paid donation of whole body while living or dead on same ground, though unpaid whole body donation while dead and not living is ethically commendable on same ground. So crux of the debate is "money matter", and really money matters for many altruists and non-altruists. Pure altruistic donation may be thus ethically cursed if and only if whole body is spiritual in nature or a gift of God who did not allow gifting it to others perhaps (and we know all this, strangely!).

Some antagonists are of the opinion that deliberate transfer of organs at some cost only apparently does not affect the whole body, but the truth is that it does affect the whole because the more and more we treat parts of our body as means to earn, our perception of the value of the whole changes gradually. We start thinking that the whole of me is saleable. This is the *slippery slope argument* – a gradual slip to an unethical limbo. At this state of a society full of such slipped persons, selling oneself at any cost or a vegetative person or a brain dead or cadavers will be unlivable. Can human life be more or less undignified? But such futile imaginations hold good in an ideal uncivil state bereft of positive laws and enforcing functionaries who least control practices of wrong trade on organs. In a civil state, which is law abiding, another perception of human dignity might evolve, and that is, reasonable trade in organs is for the greater good. Still one might argue that the open ended trade allows penetration of malpractices and also the possibility that there may be no trade at all in highly civil states. The question is: did we evolve as highly ordered humans whose rational self has transcended the limits of "earning" in "donating" ?

Antagonists have some more arguments. They hold that commoditization and thus *monetary relation* between the donor and the recipient destroys the intimate social relation, the bond so needed for a civil society to exist for long. Monetary based organ transfer divides the society from within, people treat one another as competitors in the market and a feeling of hatred grows in recipients who did not have least sympathy at worst time to do some monetary favour. The protagonists hold that in market situations, no transaction amounts to such hatred and divisiveness if it did, human society would have perished long ago. Here the point is whether or not donor-class exploits recipient-class, if there is some check and balance, no exploitation could lead to a struggle or even hatred. Many antagonist also argue that sale of body parts is mainly due to lack of funds for prolonged costly treatment, at times to meet huge debts, which might thus lead to catastrophic organ sale on the part of the person in debt. It is also possible to transfer some such materials which should not have been sold. Here again protagonists would argue that all these things happen in an anarchic state where law and its enforcement has taken a back seat.

Given these arguments and counter-arguments regarding organ donation at some cost or commodifying them, we can say that a middle path could be seen here, which holds that *unpaid donation* along with *restricted paid donation* or *limited donation* of parts and products of body might be ethically desirable in modern world in which many people are waiting anxiously for a fresh lease of life. The decision of payment or free lunch in organ transfer is a matter of donor's decision, recipient's status and abilities and control of the state in which transaction goes on under legal vigil. On the basis of this middle way to partly allow commoditization as and when deemed to be essential, one comes to consider whether or not human *reproductive materials* need to be commoditized and transferred. It is important to notice in this regard that though selling reproductive services are ethical-legal, much unethicality and illegality go with sale of gametes or germ cells. It has been objected that its sale is highly unethical because that amounts to selling a person. In fact, gametes are half way to a fully grown person and its trade amounts to not only dangerous sale in life itself but also have serious effects on demographic patterns. The protagonists however say that gametes are in no way half-way-to-life, because only zygotes contain full information of life. Hence, the point of selling person is not good. Antagonists argue that selling gametes exploits a poor woman for their eggs in an unethically constructed market of children by fixing high prices for male reproductive materials on the ground of higher biological value, though this situation is still not visible, we should notice that such a situation may be affectively countered by law and its enforcement and avoid the situation, says the protagonists. But the problem is, should we commodify zygotes, which we believed to be potential persons containing necessary biological information and genetic identity? Certainly, unlike gametes, zygotes merit some ethical concern because well decided sale of such material amounts to sale of persons in a market vulnerable to wilt under any pervert pressure. Most important is that the structure of the society allowing zygote trade might well allow whole of human being on sale if needed for money. This is a very complex market situation not to be easily controlled by law and enforcement because much depends on the traders' own ethical perception of children and adults. The traders would love to deal in zygotes fitting the greatest demands of a national and international market again damaging demographic patterns as well as human dignity. The only excuse left for the protagonists in this situation is to say that trade in such things is too premature and before any menace hits, we should be able to *restrict* zygote sale to exceptionally urgent or unavoidable cases approved by law or else we have to give up paid donation or sale in this case at least.

The greatest problem we now face is about *commoditization of genes or of genomes*, which, unlike gametes and zygotes, are non-spatio-temporal realities as much as software representable in biochemical or linguistic terms. At best we can compare these to our *intellectual property*, which reveals structure of potential life, and as such may be legally safeguarded for sale by a person, group of persons or agencies for earning something out of the deal. However, people argue that such properties are owned universally and thus does not guarantee sale by one party and not another. Rather the sale may not be allowed at all. However, the problem is that already some biotechnological companies have genetically engineered mice and patented them for sale in term of intellectual property. It is quite likely that to patent a genetically engineered human being for sale for huge profit amounts to the same as commodifying whole of human being and threaten respect for life. The human buying and selling in this way, as if, Edison has sold blueprint of one of his inventions is serious because in the world market only those dominate in such transaction whose purchase power is best and the purchaser could be at whims to use the know-how. It all comes to the perception of modern man, about the way he considers life, human beings and intellectual properties. The matter is simply not to be restricted by some laws or deterrence. Arguably free and unrestricted sale of genome needs to be under close ethical scrutiny, and it is generally assumed that biotechnological companies need to be under the scanner of global perception of human life. There must be some talk about why such genetic mapping is needed and why the property should be transferred. In any case, it would be over-simplistic to argue that all reproductive materials stand good possibility of free trade on ethical grounds.

An interesting point that has emerged in the discussion about paid donation versus unpaid donation is that though in principle unpaid donation amounting to elevated altruism appears to be good enough, it is also true that even if the donor was too good a person to do some selfless act, nothing comes as free-lunch in practice. Further, though pure altruism is so good ethically speaking, reasonable egoism and self-fulfilment is not egotism of gross variety so as to label it 'unethical'. These points and some others emerge violently in the debate of paid versus unpaid donation of human blood for therapeutic purposes. It would be however, a little too much to argue about the ethic of donating blood but there were (and perhaps are) views about equating such acts with deliberate harm to human health. It is not uncommon in India among many so-called educated people to believe that donating blood is as good as foolishness, inviting weakness and loss of strength. Yet, with growing menace of deadly infections through blood, we are more apprehensive about careless blood donation at least if not about blood donation itself. Apart from the arguments about compulsory tests during donation and post-donation care, and many intricate matters related to blackmail, we are now poised to concentrate more on paid *versus* unpaid donation as far as their respective ethical desirability is weighed. Those who strongly support the ethical desirability of voluntary, unpaid donation of blood and plasma mainly base their argument on an ethical first principle called "altruism" which propagates the idea that ethically desirable acts need to be some such human voluntary acts which "maximizes good over evil of moral agents all over the world". It is broad enough to hold that moral agents should not be differentiated according to their caste, creed, nationality, and faith and so on. It is still broader to include non-human animals or even the entire ecological community but we may restrict altruism to moral agents without much fuss. Now pure altruism does not allow any value to pure egoism, it only speaks of good for moral agents other than me. However, many "altruists" feel shy about such headstrong ethics because maximization of good for all moral agents in the world is not possible without some good for me. How can the world flourish when there is no good for me? Why will it be sensible to keep myself in pain always and maximize good for others? Hence, rationally speaking, when we speak of altruism as an acceptable ethical principle, we speak of an ethical theory which speaks of maximization of good of people other than me primarily and also the same for me to an extent that does not contradict or is not adverse to my primary goal in life, rather, in accordance with it. If we allow this, perhaps there is no "pure altruism" at all. We rather conceive of "altruism" in a qualified sense. It is interesting to notice that we have successfully rejected the ethic of "asceticism" and "rigorism" which theories in connivance with "pure altruism" have become unacceptable. Popularly, Indian ethics, particularly the Jaina ethics faces the charge of such foolhardy pure altruism amounting to asceticism and rigorism, but that is a gross misunderstanding of Jaina literature. We shall stress that any logical and rational ethical system is hardly "pure altruistic". However, if we are in need of naming an ethical theory that propagates the idea of relatively greater or primary or more broader good of human beings rather than that of me, we may use "altruism" for that theory.

Apart from many ethically desirable aspects of donation of human blood such as its being cheaper for the recipients irrespective of their purchase powers, it is argued that it is ethically desirable in so far as it promotes altruism and thus enhances social solidarity. This view has been mainly encouraged in our times by Peter Singer, Titmuss and

Keown. These forceful views have been refuted by both the supporters of voluntary paid donation of blood and 'altruism leading to social solidarity'. What the protagonists of 'altruism leading to social solidarity' have in mind is that with Singer we can believe that altruism is good itself and it grows when we become so, that is, when we go on doing altruistic acts as per habit and when many people of such character go on increasing. This amounts to the evolution of a moral state of society which makes us stronger from within than remain moral islanders. When it comes to unpaid donation of blood, the proponents of this view holds that voluntary act of donating blood for the good of others at no cost, sidesteps egoism, egotism, monetary interests etc. It is, therefore, an act purely for the sake of others whereby I draw no good for myself or that which is "altruistic". Presuming "altruism" itself as ethically desirable or good, it should be a *social policy* to encourage such altruistic donation of blood because in doing so, society gains "solidarity", which is good itself. Hence, both "altruism" and "social solidarity" being bases of ethical goodness, unpaid blood donation is good as well and thus to be encouraged as a social policy.

The antagonists of this theory such as Hugh V. McLachlan argue that an act that is "unpaid" such as donating blood, is not itself altruistic act necessarily. There is no logically necessary relation between "unpaid act" and "altruistic act" because we can find instances of some paid acts which are altruistic. Hence, even if blood donation is at no payment, it is not necessarily altruistic because the blood donated may be corrupted, unusable, unsuitable and even donated for self esteem or pity or mere sympathy or good name or gain or even to harm people. Hence, by the face value of non-payment to the donor, the value of donors' act as altruistic cannot be judged. Further, the sweeping assumption that "altruism" is good-itself is unacceptable because we can show that in the garb of such act, an agent wanted money or fame or pride or post and position. We can also assume that one who has no care for own good and good of his kin, cannot be a great saint. More interesting is to notice that a person who always places himself at last often punishes himself and his family unnecessarily for others because either the person has no moral sense or is unbalanced or a psychopath or is cunning who does everything for his good status and fortune. These people in reality cut themselves off from the mainstream of the society, their family members and friends have little regard for them or are highly disrespectful to them, and are thus divided from within. Hence, altruism does not necessarily amount to social solidarity and thus to be encouraged as social policy. It is not absurd to imagine about a person who donates blood unpaid, every month for others, are hated by many or are subjected to bad name because they do little for themselves and the family. These "selfish" people thus do no good to the society because many poor and needy people who want to donate blood for some gain are dismayed by such instances. Hence, unpaid donors' acts boomerang on other donors who nevertheless want to donate blood, serve others but not free of cost. We thus lose many more donors, rather many more than free donors. In fact, it is a poor idea that always in our societies people are selfish and they love free-lunch. It is due to this that proponents of paid donation are hailed as a morally good policy than the unpaid one. It attracts more donors, especially those having rare groups but is needy or thinks that nothing should be free of cost if it is so valuable and good. Moreover, as we have seen before, nothing really is free when we donate blood for the recipient. Why should then all others make merry at the cost of the donor? We must realize that the interested donor needs a thorough pathological check-up needing some money, they should be provided some health drink after donation which is not free, the process of blood collection need some infrastructural facilities which is not free and at times the donors should be brought from a distance involving some money (for bus fare and so on) because they cannot afford that. Who has to ultimately pay for all these things? Certainly the recipients who are not necessarily poor and needy, and even if they are, health care cannot be *completely* subsidized or better should not be subsidizes if public exchequer's health is to remain good for long.

The protagonists to voluntary unpaid blood donation argue that their position is either not properly understood or is distorted by the antagonists. First, they never suggest that all should follow the suit of unpaid donation as an imperative or that government should have certain checks on paid donation. They simply suggest that certain human acts should be for the good of the mass and not for a class, and if we believe the importance of this, societies not full of wealthy people come to realize that for a number of people something should come at a *low cost* at least, if not completely free. Granted that donation of blood is related to money, we just cannot avoid it but in principle we should accept that at least by not paying to many donors, we minimize the cost of the product, which is thus cheaper to many needy and poor. Further, altruism is certainly one strong basis for donation of blood or else why should even beggars donate blood to earthquake and disaster victims when that life saving material is so needed? Is it not true that at one point of time in the world bulk of blood, rare ones inclusive, is needed and at that time the wealthy fail to get it. Moreover, protagonists hold that among other ways, unpaid blood donation policy with a strict vigil for quality does encourage fringe donors who do not donate blood for they are not properly educated about its social value. Truly, the protagonists never attempt to suggest that private blood banks should be abolished or paid donors should be stopped donating blood, rather when it comes to relative weighing of paid and unpaid donation of this life saving material, they argue that more unpaid donation is ethically speaking, more valuable, though we must remember that many things are ethically more valuable but as is the prevalent culture in different societies, pragmatic value of something not so ethically desirable at the present epoch outwits it, but that is not a testimony to the fact that only that practice is desirable or universally good or shall remain pragmatically valuable at another epoch.

Many things have been said about organ transplantation, transfusion, banking and donation. The ethical questions and debates in particular incite us to propose our view. Now let us do a "thought experiment". Let us conceive two worlds, one in which people believe that bioethical-talk is sensible enough but it is none of our business to 'participate-and-find' how resolutions to bioethical problems are possible and what should be done in the future, and another world in which people believe that ethical-talk is not mere talk rather it amounts to 'participate-and-find' how bioethical problems should be resolved and what needs to be done in future. Certainly, one would prefer living in the second world because there we do not live in tension nurturing many ethical crises or even we do not live in inaction thinking that theoretical concerns are sufficient and resolving crises are matters important to the health caretakers and/or ethicists provided they perform certain "theoretical" tasks in isolation. Hence, we prefer a world where there are at least some people who believe that reading bioethical literature – a gamut of tricky theory, debates and so on is not sufficient enough because value-laden biomedical crises needs serious effort on our part to actively participate in *ethical dialogues* and find out ways to resolve crises and subsequently frame decision-making rules in association not isolation. In fact, biomedical ethics, as I understand it as a branch of "practical ethics" needs apart from theoretical discussions, some active participation in ethical resolution. It is very interesting to notice that many debates and questions we have seen in this chapter are not all good to read because reading them and becoming wiser by knowing our skill to think better is not pragmatic enough. What is needed on our part is to apply our ethical knowledge which is not merely knowledge of what has been passed on to us as true but what we logically justify as ethical to resolve some crises in biomedicine by discussing these things with many interested parties. Wise bio-ethicist who have read this book or such other literature are themselves unethical moral islander if they are mere onlookers of what goes on around them. Let us accept that our theoretical churning does not convince anyone why Xenografting is ethical unless we face situations of strong moral disagreements and agreements which present us newer ways of consensus, and, therefore, ethical ways to decide about trifling matters.

Readers must be aware by this time that I am hinting towards "intersubjective corroboration" about Xenografting as an ethical problem or else the number of protagonist and antagonistic views leads us nowhere. Still we should be careful about selecting parties. Certainly the surgeons, those having experience of transfer of biological materials, Xenograft experts, patients receiving or waiting to receive biological materials, lawyers and other interested parties make a good group to discuss about such matter. However, to start with, we may include views of experts in transfer of human organs (including blood) if Xenograft experts are not available for debate. The recipients' views may be concealed on request or presented in a debate in their absence after talking to them separately because most of the time they do not come up to participate in a discussion. Other things necessary for such dialogue is (as we have seen), well constructed Questionnaire prepared carefully by an ethicist or bio-ethicist after applying his theoretical wisdom as well as his experience of talking to the selected or unselected participants at the initial preparatory stages of a dialogue. The theoretical debates in this book and elsewhere for instance, is one good aid to know which question should be put to our participants but we have to talk to them personally and must have first hand idea of what people think about such matters. Next there is on card a grueling debate which should be conducted with all wits to channel a consensus and not cacophony so that our professionals are presented with a set of rules for decision-making having an ethical face. In the early months of 1999, I have talked to a number of physicians, lawyers, patients and others about this matter to select following participants for the dialogue: Dr. Majid Alam, Professor of Surgery of the then RMCH (now RIMS), Ranchi, Dr. B.P. Kashyap, Ophthalmologist and expert in cornea transplant in Kashyap Eye Hospital, Ranchi, Dr. Rajat Ray, Professor and Former Head of Surgery in RMCH, Ranchi and Dr. M.S. Bhatt, Professor of Surgery in RMCH, who took great interest in medical law (Dr. Bhatt has retired now after chairing the department in RIMS and is now a qualified Lawyer). The Questionnaire is given below:

QUESTIONNAIRE

1. Why are humans and non-human animals valuable to you? What kind of a relationship should be treated as ethical among humans and non-human animals?
2. What 'rights' should we enjoy over our biological bodies including all biological materials when we are living or we are dead? Do you think that we have some duties towards other beings, biological materials being means to perform those duties?
3. Do you think that it is morally desirable to donate biological materials we possess even though others may not be so benevolent to us? Would you prefer free donation, if yes, what is your prescription about paid donation?
4. Is it ethically justifiable to fix conditions for transferring biological materials we have donated? Who has the moral authority to decide and control over methods of donation, banking and transfer of biological materials?
5. In view of what has been replied to the first question, kindly assess your view about killing animals for organ transplants. Is it ethically desirable to clone animals for subsequent Xenografting? Is it ethically desirable to clone humans for organ transplants?
6. Kindly suggest some decision-making rules for an effective and ethically viable organ donation, banking and transplants as well as for transfusion of blood and plasma.

Dr. Majid Alam thinks that the "value" of humans and non-human animals lies in their "usefulness" in this biotic society and for the advancement of sciences. Hence, for Dr. Alam animals in general are valuable as means towards the sustenance of biotic life and advancement of scientific knowledge. He thought that living man being the most developed species in the evolutionary history is certainly of greater biological value as well as other practical value than many non-human animals and dead humans; their *well-being* is supreme. Rather, "wholesome welfare" (biological inclusive) in the *highest end* of human life for which the "use" of other humans, non-humans and dead humans in a rationally justifiable but not in ecologically harmful ways should be good enough conceivable "relationship" among the living and the dead entities in the world. Dr. Alam emphasizes that all living humans enjoy exclusive rights over his entire biological existence that includes all organs and products and even the dead state of the body provided in the last case, he or she has a registered will or a well-documented proof of his or her wish about how cadaver should be "used". Dr. Alam does not believe that any other natural or supernatural entities have any right over a person's body and all its organs and thus cannot dictate what should be done with it while living or dead, though suggestions for rational use leading to human welfare is always welcome. He holds that our "duty" as a responsible social being is to donate those materials while living in a reasonable way when it is deemed to be necessary to other humans. Even the cadaver in totality ought to be used when deemed to be necessary for the highest good, that is, "human well-being". It is also "desirable" in so far as it amounts to growth of scientific knowledge. Dr. Alam was emphatic in rejecting the value of any religious notion, that is, both the idea that organs should not or should be donated while dead or alive on supernatural dictates or favours or fear. No prejudices and commands about last rites should be thus allowed because any cadaver of a person who was living erstwhile should either have the wish to allow it to use or to destroy it, or else, rational beings in society should act rationally in favour of human welfare to do the best in cases of unavailability of written will or spoken wish. This allows us to say that "unconsented use" of organs of cadavers for the higher goal stated above, should be ethically allowed at times because it is the best (practical) use of the otherwise living person having a social responsibility.

Dr. Alam says that for him "free riding" in case of organ donation is a repugnant idea because when holistic welfare of mankind is in question, one should not enjoy all biological benefits free of cost though he is least ready even to donate a drop of blood when necessary. On the other hand, freely sharing our organs as well as blood is ethically desirable for that allows human welfare. Not only this, if the higher ideal is kept in mind, in the noble act there should be no talk about paid organ donation or paid blood donation – free sharing should be also free of cost. The simple reason is that when we adore an altruistic act which is not against ourselves as well, when we care for humanity at large, we cannot bring self interest, self esteem, gains and benefits in it. We should not unnecessarily care who has money or who has not because "money" in this case, that is, in biological welfaristic act like "donation" is secondary. Still worse, thinks Dr. Alam is to fix "conditions" for transfer of biological materials after donation and banking, that is, to fix who should get which material I have donated. Again the simple reason is that when the higher ethical ideal is at stake (and if we really value it), our decisions for transfer of donated materials need to be for the benefit of the people and not for myself because there is no point in using my organ by donating it to my close associates, it should be rather "open", "for any one who needs it". Selection of receivers would be thus "closed" and "bossing from the top" avoided because these are unethical in view of holistic human welfare. It is due to such bossing that organ donation through covenant and bargain becomes unethical. Organs are for humanity, human benefits being supreme, there is no ethicality in kin selection. Exactly due to these reasons and due to some possibility of egoism, favours, malpractices, unethical selections or emotional choices, donation, banking and transfer of biological materials should be under the strict control of the qualified health care professionals, particularly the physicians. Not only this, physicians and scientists should be bestowed this duty with exclusive rights on the selection for material transfer as ably governed by not a person or a small group but by responsible board of non-profiteering people because such method needs care for "rejection phenomenon" and "transmission of diseases" apart from subtle politics and use of money and power. A collective is thus better placed in countering unethical practices. However, Dr. Alam is of the opinion that with regard to organ donation and organ transplantation *consent* of the donor and proper *information* are both important. This is to say that the donors and the receivers in principle enjoy every right to acquire necessary biological or scientific information about why donations and transplants are needed and what if any are the post-donation and transplantation risk factors. With this necessary information, the donor and the receiver should both consent to donation and transplantation. This is ethical in so far as consent and information sidesteps malice, bluffs, misguidance, exploitation and cunning in the whole process of donation and transplantation. It makes the process more open to public scrutiny as well so that some ethical check is also on the health care professionals as well. In case of a donor becoming too critical and does not leave a documented will or wish or at least instruction to close people, in the name of public welfare, it is not a good ethical means to take decision to terminate life or extract organs at the critical state or form cadavers because physicians and scientists need not be taken as people beyond social rules and laws who have their own ways to do things. Moreover, whimsical decision-making or acting as per isolated decisions may be motivated by some ulterior gains or malice, which should be guarded in such cases. Though saving a life is important, no disrespect should be there towards freedom of choice and decision of the most important party, the donor. Equally true is that coercive or compulsive or bluffed transplants on receivers are not good means to achieve the end of well-being.

Dr. Alam has been extremely careful in maintaining that biological well-being of human beings is the highest good, Xenotransplantation is certainly an ethically permissible *means* irrespective of transplantation of animal organs of pigs or whatever. He holds that there should be no religious or emotive fixity in our minds about using such and such animal organs for human cure and care. However, before such transplants, sophisticated and careful experiments on animals should be conducted knowingly fully well that in the process some animals had to die for the sake of human well-being. Dr. Majid clarifies at this point that looking at the fragile ecological balance and the poor state of some animal species, we should be very careful about selecting pigs or baboons for ruthless Xenotransplants. It would be better that we avoid live extraction of organs of threatened species or should have back up cloning technology available to us for procuring needed organs for humans. Cloning of most suitable animals for most urgent cases of transplants is thus one good way to human welfare. Humans beings being at the helm of existence we should use animals in a judicious way, i.e., not threatening biotic imbalance, but for all this cloning should be a wider practice as well as affordable or else

Xenotransplants are themselves distant dream. Hence, Dr. Alam emphasizes Indian Law to accommodate necessary cloning and Xenotransplants in this country and for that reason it would be too harsh on scientists to penalize them on fictitious grounds. However, Dr. Alam was equally emphatic on the point of the unethical use of animal organs for private gains that is to treat them as commodity by a scientist or a group of people or an institution or organization. In any case when welfare is the point, monetary value is only secondary in the process of organ transplantations. Hence, organs of humans and non-humans should be treated as private property or property of a class to have maximum gains. What it amounts to is that in Xenotransplants and human to human transplants, though money is involved, we should have effective mechanism to check the spirit of business, profits and flourishing trade in organs which is against the ideal of biological well-being of all classes of suffering people. This would amount to minimizing costs of extraction, donation, banking and transplantation as nothing like this could be provided completely free of costs. Still control over commoditization and profits is extremely important, otherwise it would certainly be beneficial only for the affluent class. The same holds good in case of materials like blood and sperms. For Dr. Alam, donation of vital organs like kidney and cornea as well as materials like blood, plasma and sperms should come from donors who do not fix a price for it, whether the price is lower or higher does not matter much, what matters is to put some checks in inflation of the cost of Xenografting, transplants, transfusions and banking etc. at all important points. Certainly, if we need to take the help of private houses who provide facilities for collection, banking and transfer of materials, who charge heavily for profit, at least at some point, that is, at the point of donor, the cost may be reduced. It is however, important to have more public organizations and government hospitals providing low cost collection, banking and transfer because at these places even the physicians involved in transfer of materials need not be paid heavily. All these stops and checks are ethically desirable for the good of mankind and most essential for poor nations like India. Hence, paid donation, that is, payment at the initial point to the donor (which is nevertheless avoidable), is unethical according to Dr. Alam. It appears that for him benevolence does not go along with the ideas of earning, whether the donor is poor or is well off. Yet, other unavoidable points where some amount of money is needed for all *practical purposes* or else there is no progress in transfer of materials, should be strictly checked and balanced under public scrutiny or the involvement of the government machinery. Dr. Alam finds no way to compare benevolence on the part of the donor and expenses on the part of the receiver so that all others barring the donor gains, because at post-donation stages everything "practically" does not come at free of cost. Nevertheless, it is again a matter of personal feeling and ethicality to "minimize essential costs" and to "avoid the profit part either completely or radically". Dr. Alam does not think that donation, banking and transfer of sex-related materials like sperms should be tagged to the concepts of "selection for better progeny" and "selection of receivers" because these things are against the basic idea of biological welfare of mankind. Dr. Alam has some reservations about avoiding the practice of "adoption" in case of childless couples and going for very costly reproductive techniques for a child because the practice may not be doing any good to the helpless and the bereaved orphans. Yet, he mentions that affordable transfer of reproductive materials cannot be trashed as unethical for this reason because apart from growth of scientific expertise, it does give happiness to childless couples, and is thus welfaristic to some extent. Dr. Alam suggested certain rules for transfer of biological materials to which we shall come at the end of analyses of the views of all the participants.

Dr. B.P. Kashyap had no differences whatever regarding the basic positions of Dr. Alam. He dittoed that in the nature, humans, animals and other living beings are in a homogeneous relationship though for existence one heavily depends on others. In this scenario it would be ethically desirable for the most evolved species, that is, man to strive for own good and the good of the entire life-world. Hence, we may say that ethically speaking, for beings it is desirable to act in accordance with the ideal of well-being of the entire natural existence. However, when we speak in biomedical parlance, we may say that even our ideal is to strive for the biological well-being of the entire human race, which may be in one sense within the greater ideal of "well-being of the nature on the whole". Hence, for a physician it is ethically primary to ensure biological good of persons of any nation, caste, creed and faith. Dr. Kashyap was as emphatic as Dr. Alam to stress on the exclusive personal rights of human beings over their body and for that matter enjoying all rights to ensure the way whole of his body or parts therein should be used after death. Rather, it is the social responsibility of a person to decide sanely while alive about the fate of his precious biological materials. Hence, as humans our duty is to ensure maximum good of other needy persons with whatever biological gift we have. In this matter there should be no intervention of the state and religion. However, it is the state and the public to see whether or not biological materials have been used properly without any abuse, particularly without monetary gamble and blackmail. Dr. Kashyap thinks that we should not depend on contrary examples of people, who do not donate their organs for a higher purpose, we should remain faithful to our wisdom and ethical sense. Hence, it is our rationality that calls for unpaid donation (on the part of the donor) without caring who does what with his or her organs. In this sense, free donation is ethically good and paid donation not a commendable idea because benevolence does not come at cost, whatever is the monetary status of the donor. Certainly more unethical idea is to live in society as persons on crutches, that is, to free-ride on benevolence though not contributing even a little in biological terms. Sometimes we are physically not in a position to donate any organ but we use some organs donated by others, which is different altogether from egoistic free-riding of able persons. Society needs good biological education to cope up with this ignorance about value of free donation to save many lives, which is itself a noble idea, no amount of money can replace it. Dr. Kashyap agrees that if our free donation of organs is truly benevolent, it is for the greater social good, we have no ethical right to boss over the physicians to select particular persons for transfer of the donated material. There should be no will or wish like that because only the physician knows best how organs are to be used safely. At this point Dr. Kashyap showed me many newspaper cutting and photographs of poor and well-off people who had selflessly donated their cornea without any precondition, be it money or favour or selection of recipients. However, he says that physicians face many difficulties when they go for cornea collection or collection of donated parts after death. There are instances when he and his wife (Dr. Bharati Kashyap, cornea transplant expert) were called at late night or in wee hours by sensible people who knew that the person who died had pledged cornea to our eye bank (private), and we have to go there, face a lot of trouble collecting donated organ from the deceased body owing to emotional outburst of family members. Hence, doctors ought to play the role of biological counsellors. Dr. Kashyap thinks that person responsible for transplantations should try to be good counsellors, and make effort to minimize the operational and post-operative expenditure so that the receivers are also at some benefit. In fact, expenditure is one crucial factor in the success of organ transplantation which needs to be curbed. Dr. Kashyap differs to say that the private institution have great role to play in this regard. Apart from good infrastructure, trained personnel, dedication and honesty these institution can lessen the burden of government with regard to shortage of organs. However, he thinks that if private transplantation clinics do not do the job with some moral accountability and do not curb the ideal of profit-making, they are utter failure. Dr. Kashyap thinks that in any case, organ transplantation in India, which is, still facing a lot of challenges from religious orthodoxies and prejudices, should be continued with dedication and at a low cost but that does not amount to say that treating physicians are not worthy of getting some happiness out of their act.

It was very difficult to distinguish Dr. Rajat Ray's ethical vision from those of Dr. Alam and Dr. Kashyap regarding the six important questions about transfer of biological materials. Only interesting difference Dr. Ray made is that according to him the idea of human cloning is ethically *unacceptable* if that amounts to subsequent therapeutic use as in organ transplants. He was far less ambiguous than Dr. Alam and Dr. Kashyap about religion because he came out sharply against the idea that religions do not allow us to donate our body after death for biological use. He emphasized that if religion is antagonistic to this idea, it is anti-human and anti-welfare and thus is shunned. It is needed for donor and receiver to overcome religious bigotry to donate and receive organs for general biological good.

Dr. M.S. Bhatt did not have any major differences either with the three physicians. However, it is important to present some of his important opinions. According to Dr. Bhatt all organs of an organism have evolved to maintain survival of organism. In this course of evolution there are some organs essential for the existence of life such as heart, lung, liver, kidneys and so on. Nature has thus provided tremendous reserve for those organs which are under continuous strain such as liver and kidneys. Kidney has got 75per cent reserve so that if half of it functions properly, an organism sustains life. Parallel to this story of evolution of human and non-human organs is the story of journey of human beings from jungles to dwelling and from animals to the present wisdom thus giving us a social status. Nevertheless, our urge to remain as social beings does not prevent us from enjoying optimum pleasure as all other organisms hopefully deserve, but all this cannot be achieved by solitary existence. Only a strongly tied social existence breaking the barriers of caste, creed, race, religion and nationality can give us the most *desirable end of life*, which is *optimum pleasure and happiness* which need not be gross though. Dr. Bhatt made it very clear at the outset as did Dr. Ray that imagining a Higher Self who has created us or presented us valuable life and the realization of which Self is end of our life, are all imaginations of disappointed human beings – they are not rational. Dr. Bhatt holds that so far as a person is living, he has every moral and legal right to enjoy his body judiciously under socially acceptable ways and thus desire for the desirable happiness in life and it is expected that when he has lived this life of quality, he should donate whole of his body for scientific-therapeutic purposes. Hence, he does have the right to donate his body while he is alive through a will or a wish. It is interesting to notice here that not in complete agreement to some of the speakers, Dr. Bhatt maintains that though donation of organs is exclusively personal while living, it is not so when he is dead and left no clear instructions or its use. In such cases donation of part or whole of cadaver should be subjected to *social rules or law* because the deceased no more consciously enjoys the body though some other living associates for their happiness are heavily in need of the organ or organs. The society as such being so kind to him in his life long enjoyment should have the moral right to sanction donation. It is a pity, therefore, that customs, religion, prejudices and orthodoxy and immoral ways of thinking and showing emotions become adverse to the general happiness in society. Dr. Bhatt thinks that, therefore, there should not be a single free-rider in human society – we need to have potential willing donors or else in case of cadavers, social sanctions are needed for extraction of organs for scientific use and thus for social good. It is due to this that no donor should be allowed to donate organs when living or when dead as per his selection of candidates because that reveals his narrowness of mind, which is unethical. If happiness is so dear to him and his family, why should he not think that it is dear to humanity as such? Dr. Bhatt says that our understanding of biological evolution and balance in nature enable us to say that there is absolutely no unethicality in the judicious and rational use of non-human animals because in nature we do depend on each other. This amounts in reality to most appropriate ethical use of our scientific evolution. However, the practice of live extraction need not be whimsical. Dr. Bhatt emphasizes on the basis of his notion of ethicality that monetary value should never replace organ value, meaning thereby, paid donation at the point of donor. Organs should be thus above economic barter, and this enables him to support free donation of all biological materials possible to be used for human pleasure. Dr. Bhatt has already clarified that members of society and the legal authorities both have right to intervene in the matter of transfer of biological materials, and, therefore, the practice should be checked and balanced by social authorities.

It was extremely interesting to learn from these experts what medical fraternity in India could possibly say about ethic of the transfer of biological materials. Let us first come to the basis of the broad consensus we had just seen.

Transfer of biological materials should be under strict public vigil and needs to be widely practiced by the Public Health Organizations (PHO) and if necessary by the Private Organizations under tight legal frame and follow up vigil. (All participants)

Any Public or Private Hospital not fully equipped with latest amenities for collection, banking and transfer should not be allowed to take partial or unpragmatic ventures in this field. (All participants)

Any person needing transplant should be registered with full details and data necessary for the purpose in a National List of PHO. (Bhatt)

PHO should make available centers or prepare such hospitals at least two in every state in two different areas, which should have easy transplantation facilities. PHO can hire private hospital facilities for this purpose if needed. All such centers should be connected through internet. (Bhatt)

Live donation should be done under the strict vigil of Law available to India. True laws in India are good enough to restrict malpractices, but cadaver donation is preferable over live donation once the practice of donation of organs after death gains much momentum. (All)

Cadaver donation at present should not be imposed on us rather there should be wide biological, ethical and legal education supported by apt counselling by physicians and others. Donated bodies or organs need to be property of PHO who should find out match following the first registration, first service as well as gravity of situations. (All)

Private hospitals might do this as well provided they are equipped and under strict public scanner. (Kashyap)

Only hospitals having extremely swift action taking unit for transfer of materials such as kidneys etc. should be allowed to do the job. (All)

It is extremely important to mention here that in different parts of our country and in other countries different people might argue differently and might have other set of rules. Hence, intersubjective consensus and rules found are never absolute, they keep on changing, but every time we get them through a morally justifiable model of dialogue and not merely through wise theoretical churning of some people. It is thus open for any of us to contribute to this huge continuing process so that our society gets ethical rules for vital matters. A good example is that the Indian Council of Medical Research issued new guidelines on transfer of biological material in 1998 which has apart from those mentioned above these important features which must have come through such dialogue and consensus—(a) All institutions undertaking transfer of human materials need not take the sanction of the ICMR; rather they need to keep the council *informed* about the steps taken. (b) No research on biological materials should be conducted in collaboration with any foreign institute.

Interesting also is to notice that in case of no payment at the point of donor does not rule out incentives and International Transportation Society in 1985 explicitly stated that paying donors some compensation such as for time off work, child care, medical expenses etc. are ethically just to provide. Similarly, some incentives mostly monetary or otherwise may be given initially until the act of donation does not get a fillip.

Now we believe that much has been said and done about transfer of biological materials, the value-questions pertaining to it, resolving them and to find out decision-making rules for our professionals. Yet, an ethicist or a bioethicist is still left with arguments in a dialogue. This is extremely important because without it there is hardly any knowledge of application of ethical theories and principles. I do not believe that any of our participants in the dialogue knew anything about egoism, egoistic hedonism, utilitarianism etc. though the analysis of their ethical opinions reveal clearly that they championed two ethical theories in the main – *biological welfarism* and *hedonic altruism*—the former supported by Alam and Ray, the latter by Bhatt. However, it is more appropriate to say that Kshyap's view comes within the broader fold of altruism because for him biological well-being of human beings is not an end in itself rather means towards the higher end called "hedonic altruism" because what Kashyap (and also Bhatt) have in mind is that production of or maximization of biological good for humans would amount to maximization of their *pleasures or happiness*, which is what "hedonic altruistic" ethical theory upholds. It is interesting to find that if we take out pleasures and happiness, would it be still valuable (ethically at least, to strive for general biological welfare?) The point is whether or not biological welfare is in anyway an end in itself and whether or not we can call it an established "ethical theory"? It is not clear from what our welfarist physicians have said whether or not they support the dichotomy of ethical basis of biology and medicine and a general ethical basis, an overriding principle like altruism, which is applicable in many cases other than biology and medicine. If what they have in mind is that ethical-talk about biomedical matters does not necessarily beg an ethical first principle or theory like "altruism" rather some specific ethical rule or law or code or secondary principle like "biological good" or "biological well-being", then they are partly correct because physicians without being aware of established ethical theories can sensibly talk of ethic of biological matters on a different basis. Nothing prevents us really from recognizing the value of biological welfare qua professional scientists to uphold the case of transfer of biological materials. Equally true is that nothing prevents us from recognizing the truth that "biological welfarism" is a *means* to "altruism" because in the garb of an ambiguous "welfare" our participants feel that biological welfare is nothing supernatural or spiritual and thus should not be shrouded in any ambiguity. It would then amount to a relatively disease-free, suffering-free, pain-free state of body and mind of a person who was erstwhile in utter pain. And then we perhaps come to understand as Bhatt does that the ultimate ethical basis for justifying transfer of biological materials free of cost on the part of the donor under strict public and legal vigil is to *maximize pleasure and happiness in human societies* and to minimize pain and suffering, which is "hedonic altruism". It is also interesting to notice that though our participants have clear ideas of social responsibility and duty qua health care professionals, they do not support the idea that performing professional duty for the sake of doing duty is valuable because for them welfare and/or maximization of pleasure are overreaching ethical ideals. The best part (concealed though) is that none of the participants support pure egoism or egoistic hedonism though they do not reject the notion of pleasure for individual donors, recipients and even doctors because for them biological welfare of human race and their pleasures are most important, and we know that if pure altruism is enigmatic (as I have said before), our participants roughly recognized the value of individual pleasures within broader pleasure of mankind. It is a poor idea to take "altruism" as "pure altruism" where egoism has been carefully and completely avoided. Most important is to notice that very thin differences in this debate among the participants did not prevent them from coming to a consensus and to suggest decision-making rules having ethical face.

NOTES

1. Singer, Peter, "On comparing the value of human and non-human life" in Edgar Morscher *et al.*, (eds.), *Applied Ethics In A Troubled World*, Kluwer, Netherlands, 1998, p. 100.
2. *Ibid*, p. 100.
3. Dr. David Ayers quoted in The Statesman, Calcutta edition, January 5, 2002, p. 8.
4. Singer, Peter, "On comparing the value of human and non-human life" *op cit.*, p. 100.
5. *Ibid*, p. 98.
6. *Ibid.*
7. Hughes, Jonathan, "Xenografting: ethical issues", *Journal of the Institute of Medial Ethics*, BMJ Publishing Group, 24, 1998, p. 18.
8. Father Healy quoting Pope Pius XII in the Manila Congress, 1997, and I take it from A.S. Darr's editorial in the *Journal of the Institute of Medial Ethics*, BMJ Publishing Group, 24, 1998, p. 345.
9. For details see J. Locke's *Second Treatise of Government* (eds.) C. McPherson, Hackett, Indianapolis, 1980 and R. Nozick's *Anarchy, State and Utopia*, Basic Books, NY, 1974.
10. For details see L. Andrews, "My Body My Property", Hastings Center Report, 16.5, pp. 28-38, 1986; C. Campbell, "Body, Self and the Property Paradigm", Hastings Center Report, 22.5, pp. 34-42, 1992; R. Scot, *The Body as a Property,* Viking Press, NY, 1981; M. Swami, "An Alternative to Property Rights in Human Tissue", Hastings Center Report, 20.5, pp. 12-15, 1990.

5

Intersubjective Corroboration and the Ethic of the Beginning and End of Life

At this point I would like to make a radical change in writing about bioethical issues. I must also write about reasons for making such radical change. The radical change in style is not to consider one value-laden issue as those considered in two earlier chapters by elaborating the nature of the issues, the exposition of the range of ethical problems concerning those issues and their resolution through intersubjective corroboration. Now I would like to club two most important value-laden biomedical issues for discussion. However, in the discussion I will elaborate the nature of the fresh set of problems and analyze them, but I would not go for the elaboration of the intersubjective corroboration dialogue arranged by me. Instead of it, I now prefer to construct questionnaires regarding the resolution of these issues and then leave for all interested people who are also readers of this book, to go for such corroboration dialogue to find out how it becomes useful to professionals in biology and medicine. Nevertheless, on the basis of what I have found in real life debate regarding these issues, I shall point out which ethical first principles were active in such dialogue so that others taking up this task are able to check the similarities and the differences in this regard.

Always there are reasons for clubbing some issues than isolating them in biomedical discussion. One reason is that bioethical literature based on real-life bioethical dialogues largely depends of the given socio-economic and political conditions of a particular state of a nation. I would like to emphasize that any discussion about bioethical issues in India should be careful enough to find out which issues are of utmost importance in the present social, economic and political conditions rather than giving more stress to some such issues which are more fashionable to consider or are more emotively charged or are considered by the idea that in the near future we are going to face such problems. We understand very well at the present epoch in India that value-laden issues in public health care, the management of high risk group of patients, nursing of sick persons are of great importance. Most importantly these issues are likely to rule supreme in any bioethical discussion in times to come (in India and abroad). Naturally, I had all concern for these issues to figure in this book, not leaving important aspects of these issues, including moral debate regarding them and analysis of the outcome of the debate. The same is true in case of transfer of biological materials, whether it is human to human or animal to human. If we compare these issues with those of cloning, surrogate motherhood and so on, in the Indian context, they are certainly secondary though not unimportant for us. May be in the future we would face these problems more acutely, but it is more pragmatic not to consider them as most urgent here at this point of time, though the issue may be highly problematic in the USA, the UK and elsewhere. Not exactly in this secondary category are the bioethical issues of In Vitro and In Utero experiments, abortion, euthanasia and experiments on human and non-human animals. We may say that in the Indian context these issues are *emerging* ones or that these issues are relatively more important than cloning and surrogacy, but I still believe that they are not as primarily important for us to go for broader and broader intersubjective corroboration dialogues all over India as it is necessary in cases of public health care and transfer of biological materials. We cannot doubt that relatively rapidly emerging bio-ethical issue in India is abortion because it has direct connection with extremely important issues in *population* in a country of many religions, cultures and obsessions. Hence, these issues need to be put together for our careful bioethical considerations.

Another reason is that certain problems bear ‘family resemblance’, and, therefore, needs to be clubbed for discussion. The “emerging” issues as I have mentioned above, bear a ‘family resemblance’ because they are about *beginning and end of human and non-human life*. Abortion, euthanasia involves ending human life for different reasons though much heat is generated in whether or not in abortion we do end “life” properly. Similarly, bio-medical experiments on animals amounting to ending their lives are equally a matter of ethical concern. Interestingly, ending lives may be happily discussed along with beginning lives so far as biomedicine is concerned because "beginning" human life in particular is extremely challenging for the biologists and the medical man than "ending" lives. There is no point after so many years of the advancement of biomedicine to believe that biomedicine is merely for "sustenance" of life and at best for the "enhancement" of life. It certainly faces problems regarding two unavoidable biological stark truths: beginning of life and its certain end. It will be in bad taste to say that biomedical experts are not satisfied with their living demigod status and they would like to prove them gods who creates and if needed ends as well. The "trinity" of creator, nourisher and terminator may not be a good status for our serious biomedical men for they never aim at such status, nor should they aim at such status because becoming or assuming status of gods cannot be a justifiable ethical status for a sensible educated man, who knows that *qua* man, man is good enough to be born and dead with little amount of good he does in the world that may be equally good enough for immortality. We also come to know that the ethical concerns in beginning human and non-human lives involve a lot of *experiments*. Even sustenance and enhancement of life needs a lot of experiments, which at times, amount to ending lives, particularly of animals. Hence, with ethical issues in ending lives, we should better discuss beginning lives as well.

Readers should be rest assured that I do not mean to justify that there are no more sensible and emerging bioethical issues in India, but I would not go on extending my effort in this direction at least in this book. Other writers might take up some more issues nevertheless. Hence, let us straightway consider four important ethical issues regarding beginning and ending lives. We shall first go through beginning human and non-human lives in which tricky biomedical experiments are involved, including ending some lives for beginning some more. Next, we shall consider the cases of abortion and euthanasia—two most important cases of ending human life. But for a sensible discussion on all these topics we should at the outset clarify why exactly the problem of beginning and end of human and non-human life is worth considering in general and in ethical discussion in particular. Apparently, beginning and end of biological entities having life is not problematic – it is so "natural" in existence that we hardly feel any serious problem. However, things are not as easy as they appear to us because something having some "value" on earth should be taken seriously, particularly when we come to know that value of such things are so crucial because existence itself necessarily depends on these things or else there is no existence of "nature" as we know it "now". Take this 'thought experiment': imagine two worlds, one in which humans and non-human animals are taken to possess some existential value and the other world in which they are taken to have no such value. Imagine further that in one world no care is taken about procreation because humans and non-humans have gone mad or freak or whatever leading to "no further life"; whereas in other world sane people and normal animals procreate with and without external aids. Still further, imagine that in our first world no one cares if humans and non-humans die in any manner whatever, and given their freakiness towards procreation, they do not bother for constant death; whereas in the second world, cases of death are taken as seriously as birth. At the end of this utterly simple 'thought experiment' try to answer this question: if we are not in the illusory trap of *kārmic* cycle and immortality, which world is worth living? For me, even if I fall in *kārmic* cycle (which surely I will), I would like to begin my life in the second world afresh (which I welcome) as ant, antelope or man because there my progenitors and other peers are "normal", they behave as they should and leave a message for me to live a "normal form of life", which is tantamount to "death" but not before care have been taken to defy "death" because life-value is greater than death-value in a "normal form of life". Yet, death-value cannot be robbed of its little nobleness in a "normal" world as a system like ours cannot sustain all life but no death. Hence, in the second world we still do not hanker after biological immortality because beginning of life is not possible by some such cells in which, at one stage catabolism does overpower anabolism. Yet, constant biomedical mechanisms to "replace" our organs with other newly created ones by some people might renovate us to a great extent, or else, we are replaced by our *equally fateful* "replicas", our "clones" by yet another biological mechanism. Biomedicine thus appears to be a Sisyphus cursed with constant acts for immortality, which it cannot in principle complete.

If life and death are generally important for us to be cared on earth, there must be some discipline to take such care, and for this we have the biological and the medical sciences. However, things are a little different when we raise different set of questions. Considering all worth of living in our second world, it still makes sense to ask whether or not it is morally desirable to "take human and non-human life" or enhance their death for some reasons? This question does not lose its expected sting in the face of our touted "life value" than "death value" because there are formidable "reasons" as many believe to intervene or not to intervene in death. Similarly, it is sensible to ask in our preferred world whether or not certain bio-mechanical inputs or aids or methods are at all morally desirable for beginning life? These fresh set of questions are ethical questions about biological conceptions of life and death in the "preferred world", which we call bioethical questions about "beginning and end of life". We are here to take up these interesting and sensible questions. A little reflection on contemporary status of biomedicine and its historical growth reveals that it is not esoteric coterie of philosophers who have glorified bioethical questions about life and death rather, many biomedical scientists are equally responsible in joining the foray not for a fashion or a passion rather, for pragmatic reasons which shall be revealed as we proceed. Hence, bioethical questions like these have a pragmatic value. Apart from other things, finding answers to these questions hopefully help us in making our preferred world more livable and lovable. Readers should notice that here we are not concerned about answering ethical questions about many other "non-biological" ways for beginning and ending lives as we find in mysteries and myths. We are here not interested in the ethic of God's creative act *vis-à-vis* human interventions and in the ethic of suicide and killing for self-defense. However, we are here surely interested in the ethic of beginning non-human animal life through human intervention and ending non-human animal life by virtue of human intervention because as we have already seen, they raise important questions for ethical desirability, biological desirability notwithstanding. Though it is also important (pragmatically, biologically and ethically) to talk about beginning and end of plant life, we consider them in ecological ethics. Hence, we shall leave these issues here.

There is no doubt however that there is no point in joining to discuss the ethic of beginning and ending human and non-human life if we are not sure about who is a "human being" and who is a "non-human animal" because for the sake of argument, if fetus is not "human life", there should be no point in ending life in termination of fetus, and if a cloned entity (humans inclusive) being not "naturally procreated", does not stand the description of "animal", there is no point in beginning life either. Hence, we have to find out when some entities stand good for a description of either human being or non-human animal. In fact, a number of ethical questions about beginning and ending animal lives depend on finding satisfactory answers to these questions, which are, nevertheless, not so satisfactorily available to us owing to much theoretical disputes in biology and philosophical reflections in biology. Interestingly, in the proper scientific circles, the intrusion of philosophy regarding this matter is not disliked any more for many scientists do whisk off the sensibility of *non-biological* or better said *trans-biological* descriptions of "life" of humans and non-humans. Hence, for humans, the holy grail of descriptive definition, the "nature of chromosomes in cells" as determinately different from other non-human animals, and even "nature of fetuses embodied in female humans" is not free from controversy for description of "human life" on the simple count of "chromosomes" and fetuses. One reason is that "chromosomes" apart, "human life" should be reasonably described in terms of "self awareness", which neither fetuses nor vegetative humans possess, and "self awareness" is not completely alien to or averse to biological science. However, biologists and many others argue that in so far as description of human being or non-human life is concerned, "chromosomes" are good enough when "inclusion" into a given species is important. In any case, "chromosomes" does not seem to be sufficient to include fetuses into the set of "self aware persons", a property that stirs our imagination when we "terminate" fetuses by deliberate ways, mostly provided by biomedicine. Hence, in case of humans, "homo sapiens-hood" as different from "person-hood" paves way for stirring bioethical debate about beginning and ending human life. It is Christian thinker Joseph Fletcher who took some pain to enlist "indicators of humanhood" which are in addition to "chromosome" factor which, he thinks, enable us to see why we have enough ethical reasons not to take human life. This is in accordance with what John Locke conceived of a "person", and what Peter Singer thinks is good enough for an ethical debate about taking life.

Peter Singer in *Practical Ethics* (1993) argues that if we look at the stringent or stipulative definition of "human beings" provided by the biological science, we would have hardly anything to say about the ethical nature of the act of taking life of such beings because on the nature and count of "chromosomes" one would hardly have any basis to justify why any "chromosomatic" being (to coin a new expression), other than humans, that is, belonging to another species be killed and human chromosomatic being should not be killed. If we stick to glorifying the value of human chromosomatic race and none else, it is unethical *speciesism*. Now what is expected of us is to argue that humans transcend "chromosomaticness" by virtue of other inherent properties (or even acquired ones) so that it would be hardly justifiable to take life for different so-called "non-homicidal reasons" which are ethical. Interestingly, the same may be true of non-human animals though they have such non-human properties as valuable as human properties though not similar in nature, which transcends their "chromosomaticness". It is not hard to imagine that apart from other reasons, one strong reason for not killing animals and humans is for their obvious ecological value or biotic value. But the real problem is taking life of a "likely-human" growing within a human or a human more "like vegetable" that have visibly lost some valuable transcending properties for which they were glorified so much. It is due to this that "abortion" and "intervened death" make such good cases for ethical debates. No less enthusiastic are religious men, the theologians in particular, who argue that humans have been conceived by them as "sacred" – those transcending mere "chromosomaticness" so to say. Some more enthusiastic people find that non-human animals are equally "sacred". Hence, their ethical-religious inputs are worth considering provided we are satisfied with their basic presupposition of "sacredness". More interesting is to notice that the "bundle of virtues" which are inherent in humans and non-human animals and those transcend their grossness to sacredness may be so extensive as well as powerful that it may be difficult to justify killing of such beings in any form because fetus may be viewed as equally powerful bundle of virtues which, if allowed, extends more of virtues and thus not a party to be killed. Equally true is that a person in deep coma, turned to a vegetable, may be still a bundle of virtues not perhaps in a state of extension of some more virtues but at a losing side, though not to be killed either because strangely its "grossness" which must have some link with its "chromosomaticness" needs no interference which is humane because the person has right to live a natural death. Hence, many people like to disagree with Peter and others on the point of "chromosomaticness" because this touted biologically distinguishing property of *man qua man* is not enough to argue that humans even without transcending to a more glorified "bundle of virtues" status, raises our ethical stimulus to ask: why should fetus die? And why should the nearly dead, die at our mercy? It is very difficult to forget that the "grossness" of animals, in fact, have many refined biological values for their races, and it is not necessary that all animals are good when they serve our good only. Animal "grossness" is not good for us as we Xenotransplant; it remains good by virtue of being a member of a unique species. Animal goodness is not necessarily and sufficiently a matter of human teleological judgment. Happily the argument may be extended to human race as well. Hence, without making much fuss about "humanhood", "personhood" and "animalhood", we may justify that ethical questions about "taking life" is stirring even when humans and animals are taken as "bundle of biological virtues". But there is no problem if they are considered for more values, though it largely depends on human perception about animals, mostly on a comparative basis for transcendence of biological values. There is some cunningness one feels when this "extension" relegates animals to commodities for our use, not members of an intricate biological nexus, and we feel that all should act scapegoats to champion our existential cause. One important thing to notice is that human evaluations of animals skip the truth that bereft of evaluation of "use-value" of animals they are still useful and valuable. Another point is that our enthusiastic arguments about saving animals and to protect their right to life naturally justify that first we should live and for that some non-humans should die, is grossly mistaken because 'rights people' do not have ethical right to shelve rights of animals when human life is at stake.

However, our opinions may not be liked by many people, and, therefore, ethical debate continues. One might argue that even if fetuses have chromosomatic identities, gross biological values and non-biological values and virtues as well, on several other biological, demographic, emotive reasons, killing them is justifiable ethically. Similarly, even if humans and animals, the vigorous and the vegetative, have biological and non-biological values and virtues, they still may be killed on strong ethical reasons derived from the "teleos" of human life. This, nevertheless, makes a good debate but what concerns me most is that how should we approach such debates amounting to some resolution? Not moving any further from the model proposed by me, I would still justify that on such delicate issues only participation of the concerned parties along with an ethical corroborator towards resolving crises would help us because reading and writing volumes after volumes about ethic of euthanasia or abortion or artificial procreation won't help us to the least because analyzing issues and theoretical churnings in teleology, deontology and virtue-ethics are partly useful for a handful of people who read them but not really helpful if these people do not come forward to do something concrete. We have taken this task, and here in this chapter let us leave a few questions for the readers who start acting towards resolution on their own. Let us come, therefore, to analyse of the issues of abortion, euthanasia, ending animal lives and biological researches in beginning human and non-human animal lives before questions are for dialogues. A cursory remark is needed here: I have introduced the ethical debate about "taking life" mainly but several points mentioned in this course are helpful in understanding that "beginning life" is equally stirring when it is viewed under the ethical scanner. We shall come to it immediately as case of "beginning life" draws more attention than case of "ending life", a point which I repeat here with some risk. It is interesting to notice that 'initiate' and 'beginning' are some expressions which need not be taken as "creating life". It is expected of biomedical scientists to come forward to justify why "creating life" is a challenging question in biomedicine than a relatively reasonable "beginning life" because the scientists at the working unit of life do not believe that it drops from the sky or it happens *ex-nihilo*, rather they need certain biological materials to work with so that the *beginning* of life is made possible at a highly regulated technical atmosphere, which is not "creating life". Hence, there is no point in harping about an age-old hackneyed attack on our scientists to say that they failed (and is sure to fail) in "creating life", and, therefore, science need not be boastful about their contemporary deeds (or misdeeds, say many) like "cloning", "test tube babies" and so on and think that they have become God. The point is, who on earth is worried about claiming the status of creator God, not the scientists to be very sure because that would be essentially unscientific for a scientist to claim. Hence, given the materials we can do a lot of manipulations for beginning life forms, but not create these materials at present. However, the question is, can we really ignore the possibility of artificial creation of life initiating materials? What happens if some people are really at such work? Are they acting God? Well, we really do not know what comes next? If you ask me, given the meteoric growth of biomedical science, I dare not say that something is extremely improbable. Nevertheless, I must definitely assert that the acts of beginning of life and creating building blocks of life shall face ethical scrutiny as it has been with ending life. So without bothering much for creation of life, I would like to ask, what follows in ethics about beginning of life? And our methodology to face it should be the same as before because debates are not intellectual cacophony. Most interesting fact is that we are at the verge of facing the most important question about the entire issue, that is, why on earth should ethical questions be asked about beginning and end of life? One important reason is that deliberation and follow-up action regarding beginning and ending life are not merely pragmatic affairs in biology and medicine, they are also affairs affecting entire social life by stirring concerned peoples' mind and to know why should such pragmatic things be done and not left out? The point is that scientific justifications along with justifications based on pragmatics and intellectual satisfaction are not enough because after all these have been said, a nagging problem is, what happens if something can be shown to be undesirable in social environment though those things are useful and scientifically just? That this is extremely probable in contemporary world is well known in case of euthanasia. It is not difficult to find instances of gross unethicality in this practice that has influenced law-makers to find its practitioners as guilty of murder or killing. Equally true is that the same has been justified to be ethical so much so as to frame a new law altogether to permit euthanasia in a civil state. Hence, the ethical pros and cons of euthanasia are much different from the nitty-gritty of medical science and its pragmatic arguments do influence us to take up the challenge of facing a tough moral debate for resolution or else there is no law or a change in law. The same is true in case of artificial procreation and cloning. With this we now come to consider the cases of beginning of life of humans with special reference to In Vitro research and some allied mechanisms. (Readers hopefully remember that for me problem urgently to be resolved in the Indian context is primary). Coming to the next issue of ending life, I would like to consider the cases of experiments on animals amounting to ending their life, abortion and euthanasia.

Beginning of life of human beings and non-human animals is not a fashion or an intellectual passion or to present a technological gimmick, it has emerged out of the problem of "infertility" as well as "enhancement of animal species" for practical reasons. The entire affair is involuntary in nature and does not follow the ideal of standards of having a child through heterosexual intercourse. However, infertility is not a disease; it is a state of organism needing some medical intervention or support so that some defect in the state may be overcome. Yet, some people say that intervention in infertility is medical tailoring to fit the cosmetic and emotive needs of sexually challenged people through In Vitro fertilization. Literally, In Vitro fertilization or IVF means "fertilization in glass" because eggs from mother is removed and mixed with father's sperm in a Petri dish where fertilization takes place. This medical marvel (as some say), happened as early as 1978 in England when Louise Brown saw her life come out of Petri dish in the peculiar *non-sexual* manner. The entire process does not depend on donated reproductive cells; all embryos are constituted out of parents containing their genes and later on transferred to mother's uterus where pregnancy takes place. But the process does not rule out 'donors' because either sperm cells or the egg cells or even early embryo may be obtained from sources other than those in husband-wife relationship. In case sperm and egg cells are from husband and wife, they may be further medically intervened for chromosomal tests for abnormalities; they may be stored and even donated to others and allowed to die out after conducting researches. By this time so many options are available in IVF that the wonder baby of 1978 is a history of primary technology for beginning life. Given this background we may say that IVF along with artificial insemination and surrogate parenting as artificial means of reproduction have changed our opinion about the correlation of sex and reproduction because we thought that sex without reproduction is possible but reproduction without sex is not possible, which is however, completely mistaken. Further IVF have changed our notion of "family" whether nuclear or joint because in case of sperm donor or egg donor, nothing is absurd or orthodox about asexual reproduction. Now the point is, if husband-wife relation being most important in "family", it is at all ethically acceptable to us? Or, is asexually reproduced child emotionally acceptable to us? It is not difficult to find theists in particular to argue that with IVF, the conception of *not* having a family is encountered. An unethical idea that for•sex in society, family is redundant and a child reproduced need not belong to a traditional family of husband and wife is also encouraged. The unharnessed sex in society and the consequent effects on reproduction are feared for growing immorality apart from many practical problems. Yet, protagonists of artificial reproduction like IVF trash such fears of unethicality as they have a set of arguments to show that given the curse of "infertility", IVF is ethically desirable as it is both biologically safe and maximizes good for sexually challenged people in society. With this, we believe our readers start picking up ethical cues for a lively debate. We have seen in our earlier discussions that the act of "adoption" in this regard stirs up fresh set of questions as it challenges the artificiality, the emotions and the conception of maximization of social good by aiding sexually challenged people. Naturally in case of "adoption", a viable alternative of artificiality cannot be overlooked as a challenge, and if the barrier of "my children are truly mine in the family" be surpassed, it becomes stronger. The problem is why should "my-ness" come into this matter when IVF and surrogating does not rule out "other-ness"? Do we have to believe that IVF is good if and only if in Petri dish "my-ness" is nurtured in a husband-wife biological mixture? What if any one party is not fit to give his or her "my" or "self" through biological material and does not prefer "another" one's property? Is it desirable then to prefer at least a partial "my" in participation of at least one party of family? Many people argue that everything is fine if only deserving women select progeny in asexual manner because it is they who bear the pains of post-fertilization pregnancy and birth. Even if they were sexually challenged, they still have the right to reject unfit or undesirable sperms for future property. Hence, everything is all right only if female select sperms in IVF and come out of the "patriarchic" reproduction or even "patriarchic artificial reproduction". So we have at hand a more stimulating ethical debate when IVF itself can be trashed if it is matriarchic and does allow freedom for male "donors". Still interesting is that feminists may be against IVF even if it is matriarchic leaving other choices for progeny or none of it because in any case the female will be targeted as only available harvesting field. Why should people be so worried about infertile male or female? What if females become non-harvesting fields? Is that the ethical way to look at women?

This is not all in array of ethical questions. Many people ask why is it ethical to technologically intervene in some such matters which are essentially natural to humans and not to technology. The question is who has the moral right to bring in technology in such human affairs? What on earth is wrong if somebody had no access to artificial procreation when such intervention is "against nature" and "against God"? Sharper argument is that the world's goodwill be least changed even if handful of people did not go for IVF and had children. The maximization ideal is thus completely misconceived according to these people. Other antagonists charge IVF as unethical because it is essentially harmful to the embryos and thus disparages *right-to-life*. Interestingly, in India or elsewhere

IVF has not been legally banned for it has not been proved to be anti-human or anti-social. Rather, a good reaction comes from John A. Robertson in his edited essay in Beauchamp and Le Roy's *Contemporary Issues in Bioethics* in these words: "If a law banning IVF or GIFT were passed, it would no doubt be found unconstitutional because it directly impedes the efforts of infertile married couples to have offspring, thus interfering with the fundamental right to procreate. The moral objections made by the Catholic Church, feminists and others do not constitute the compelling evidence of tangible harm necessary to justify interference with procreative theory."[1] Hence, it would be a little too much for him as well to declare IVF completely unethical and illegal. But what Robertson in his essay nicely focuses further is that the bone of contention is the "harm to embryos argument" to establish unethicality inherent in IVF because there is no way to avoid truth of implantation of embryo into the fallopian tube and subsequent problems that come to women as well as the embryo. Many people argue that the embryo has assumed the status of "human being" and, therefore, needs all care for protecting its *rights*, particularly 'to live unharm'. But embryo is likely to suffer damages in way of implantation or preservation or further experimentation. Hence, it amounts to killing life or harming right to live and, thus, unethical. Yet, the argument does not take notice of the fact that in IVF harm to embryo while implanting is a misconceived fear. Further, it is argued that as embryos hold the same status as any normal human tissue, it should be given the same rights to remain unharmed. However, in IVF it is not given the due status in cases of its experimentation. Again the advances in IVF techniques rule out this fear. Another position is that in reality embryos deserve more respect than any other human tissue because it is a symbol of life as such. Noticeably, biologists argue that though it is potentially "life", it is still not a "person" and may or may not attain "personhood" any further. However, there are peculiar ethical controversies still raging in this regard. One group argues that "personhood" does begin at the embryo-stage and enjoys human rights. The other group, though they are Christians opposing taking life of fetus in abortion, thinks that given the biological status of embryos, it is a little too much to call it "person". If this be the ethical controversy then we have to find out consensus with regard to the most crucial point of deliberate harm on embryos in case of "selection" of a few of them in IVF to avoid multiple gestation and freezing embryos until use or discard them partly or fully. In both cases we notice that in IVF, the status of embryos and ethical questions related to it hovers around "discarding" some embryos. Apart from legal prevention of treating potent human life as trash, important value questions remain to be considered seriously. We should be responsible in answering why genetic information of great value is thrown at will just for satisfaction of a few individuals? And why should we be so ruthless in disgracing something symbolic of life? These questions make sense in case of freezing embryos because freezing process is liable to damage embryos to divide further and as a result to be discarded. The protagonists argue on the other hand that damage limit in freezing is minimal and further minimized and thus not as disgraceful as discarding them. Further, at minor losses in real life, we might gain much because freezed embryo saves the infertile when it is most needed or might be useful in posthumous use in case of death of a child. However, there are intricacies in "ownership" as well in case both husband and wife die or when they are estranged without any legal aid to support their rights. Finally, if we look at many countries like India, we question about the financial viability of the IVF process. The problem is, does it suit merely the purpose of the rich or the relatively affluent class, who for their desire-satisfaction (to get "own" offspring), affords a huge cost? If that be the case, why should such technology be called ethically good for its blatant class bias? Hence, despite several biomedical supports to IVF as mentioned by writers, Robertson notices that "socially constructed attitudes about the need to overcome infertility will be a main determinant of use. Money also counts when one is seeking access to IVF. IVF shows that procreative liberty is not a fully meaningful concept unless one has the knowledge and means to obtain IVF from the best programmes, or the will to restrict its allure when its use seems excessive?"[2]

In an excellent essay in Beauchamp and Walter's edited book, Susan Sherwin argues that "the most widely accepted moral theories of our times are inadequate for addressing many of the moral issues we encounter since they focus entirely on such abstract qualities of moral agents as autonomy or quantities of happiness, and they are addressed to agents who are conceived of as independent, non-truistic individuals... we need a theory which places the focus of ethical concerns in a complex social network of interrelated persons who are involved in special sorts of relations with one another"[3]. This is extremely important because we realize that issues like IVF or test-tube babies are not so simplistic, that ethical engineering with the aid of one moral theory would resolve the range of issues we have. Hence, socially interrelated persons should find a way out of theory cooption in this regard. Sherwin thinks that this way is provided by "feminist ethics" which is theory non-co-opted. Before coming to her claim let us find out how Sherwin demonstrates the failure of moral theories in case of resolving issues in IVF. According to Sherwin, the theological ethical justification of the wrongness of IVF is based on 'unnatural' and 'artificial interruption' in God's handiwork. Paul Ramsey, for instance, argues in this fashion in some of his papers as does Leon Kass. Kass is particularly against "dehumanization" or the "objectification" of the human subject in medical intervention to initiate life because embryos are constructed out of given biological materials which are in themselves "things" and "commodities" and not bearer of a sanctified value. However, supporters of utilitarian theory reject the divine presuppositions in case of 'life' as mere superstition. Moreover, they argue that there is an element of ambiguity in the theological assertion of "naturalness" and "artificiality" because for the theists what is "natural" is at best "divinely created or designed", which, however, creates confusion. If "naturalness" is what is in space-time as things or material objects, biological-medical interference involving such things does not enable us to call it unethical. It is also not appropriate to say that in IVF practice, an embryo is bereft of "humanness" just because it has been helped to come to existence by individuals and not by God. Utilitarian like Michael Bayles in *Reproductive Ethics* argues that any act of asexual reproduction cannot be termed 'unethical' on the fictitious ground that God permitted sexual reproduction, and, therefore, only that is good. Interestingly, if God did everything about sex, He must have given the humans the power to reproduce asexually, and, therefore, good and not bad. Utilitarians also do not like theological fear about immorality pervading in society with the sophistication of artificial reproductive technology because with it grows the chances of human cloning, which is a cultural shock for us because reproduction apart from God's miracle is a miracle of love-relationship. Utilitarians hold that these ideas are again fictitious because God's plan in reproduction is not proved beyond doubt and in IVF no less 'love' could be seen between the parents. Human cloning on the other hand is not culturally shocking as with the growth of our reproductive knowledge (which is essentially biological and nothing else); this technology should be as much acceptable as any other technology which we have already accepted. Most important point is that technologies like IVF need to be *ethically evaluated* keeping in mind the exclusive consequences of the technology itself and not keeping in mind what is assumed about religious and other consequences. It is difficult here to digest that an ethical evaluation of IVF technology would be possible without considering its effects on society, culture and religious faiths. No one would deny that in India wider IVF practice would pose great problems for our law-makers when religious groups start throwing stones on them. One call may be to abolish religions, which pose greater problems at this date. Anyway we cannot sanely overlook IVF's religious repercussions in society. We have already seen that religion apart, non-religious or even atheists may debate at length about the "status of embryos". If it does show signs of human life, can we go on to produce surplus of these things and further follow a trash-bin policy? Can we treat either mother's womb as bio-garbage or throw surplus embryos if the garbage is full? In first case, mother's womb turns out to be a perfectly unmanageable piggery and in the later case, sheer disrespect for life is shown or at least products at high cost are wasted for nothing. We have also seen that these questions about IVF further drag us to the status of embryos and to the issue of *rights*. However, utilitarian in one wise stroke would justify the IVF technology as ethical in the face of all the ethical fears that everything is good if it produces a greater balance of human good in societies over evil produced. Nevertheless, some thinkers argue that things are not as simplistic as utilitarians hold because the clumsy, intricate and money consuming technology cannot be so good as to maximize human good in societies, it maximizes human good in a few cases of affluent class but that does not constitute the whole of the society. Moreover, if it is a matter of "private players" and not the "public", the motive of maximization of personal profits of handful technologists cannot be justified as socially good. Truth is that no public expenditure on such projects is visible in countries like India for the good of a section of sexually challenged people when greater health care challenges ask for heavier public expenditure. Deontologists on the other hand have a mixed bag for us as they would like to settle to use one's free and autonomous will. The technologists and the needy alike should conceive wilful agreement as most important so that on the one hand intrinsic goodness of IVF is saved from any challenge and on the other hand there is no moral scare for treating embryos as means to a personal gratification.

Sherwin remarks after a survey of these traditional ethical theories that "Feminists share many of these concerns, but they find many other moral issues involved in the development and use of such technology and note the silence of the standard moral approaches in addressing these matters"[4]. Sherwin rightly notices that a feminist moving away from the theoretical burdens of ethics would resort to newer ethical answers, for instance, *autonomy of women* in case of IVF because it is they who bear the pangs of post-implementations, and being the donor of eggs, she does have a say in it. Further, they do have freedom in choosing IVF for their good such as having children, which is so natural to a woman. Yet, it is true that autonomous women are always under the compulsions of the technology and the technologists for their good. Hence, women's 'autonomy' is partial, only in deciding to have a go at IVF but only IVF and the experts can decide whether her wish needs to be fulfilled or can be fulfilled or should be fulfilled. The situation that emerges, therefore, is that the stakeholder is at the receiving end of the mercy of the stockholder. The business goes in a head-down fashion, much at the will of the clinic who provides the service, does not let any bargain or gratis, and for sure, the poor women cannot speak in her terms of satisfaction or cannot pose a competitive threat by consulting other clinics like she would do with mobile phone services. Hence, feminists should better notice the limitation of speaking like deontologists by projecting the case of "autonomy" falsely. Similarly, a feminist should take care for the fact that there is not much to be puffed up about maximizing their good, which is so much touted by utilitarians because rather than doing their good, it may be a great threat to women's role in reproduction as success of IVF leads way to other asexual procedures like cloning where women are seriously challenged for their disposition to reproduce. And if that be true, why should liberty to produce "males only" be not a new passion? These inherent threats call for safer measures in reproductive processes.

Sherwin thinks that a new looks feminist analysis of the ethic of IVF should hit the truth of treating 'child' as a *commodity* and *personal property of women*. With these go the idea that at some cost a valuable child is *needed for women* and as such it is she who has to *care*? The vanity of women existence is *complete* by having "own baby" at some cost and suitable design artificially cannot be ruled out either. The ethical questions of women existence in relation to child and reproduction emerges in these contexts. Is it ethically justifiable that women are looked upon as cry babies who would be doomed without designer babies, the costly commodities who then become her burdensome property to nurture? Sherwin further puts a feminine assertion of caring "several babies" in this context. She says, "In such a world it would not be necessary to spend the huge sums on designer children which IVF requires while million of other children starve to death each year. Adults who enjoyed children could be involved in caring for them whether or not they produced them biologically"[5]. This is a good appendage to the criticism already noticed about the maximization theory which now appears to be a wolf of capitalist prodigality in the cloak of welfarism. Nevertheless, Sherwin is very sympathetic to couples who could not produce "their" children for biological handicaps but in the overall situation of human welfare they still have to think of other measures if needed. This may be one strong basis of "adoption" as I believe.

What Sherwin says finally is of greater interest for me because she realizes that feminists should care for a reproductive ethic in which ethical imbroglios of IVF, cloning and many more need not be merely analyzed for clear understanding and endless arm-chair debate rather find out a more "caring model to resolve these issues". What on earth could be *feminine model*, a caring one so to say, much different from the imposing patriarchic model for ethical resolution of IVF? As I understand Sherwin, she holds that a patriarchic model of resolution of issues like IVF, a matter related to female individuals, mainly needs *necessarily and sufficiently* some *ethical theories* which are unilaterally used by experts to end the said ethical impasse, which for me, is the "engineering" model. The chauvinism of experts in ethics (male or female) with imposingly true theories is thus 'patriarchic', whereas the 'feminine model' is as she says, "In my view a feminist ethics is a moral theory that focuses on relations among persons as well as on individuals. It has as a model an interconnected social fabric rather than the familiar one of isolated, independent atoms.... It is a theory that focuses on concrete situations and persons and not on free-floating abstract actions"[6]. Hence, a feminist model would prefer to consider the *resolution* of the problem of IVF in close cooperation of theory non-co-opted people, the biologists, the technicians, the parents, the donors and many more so that IVF does not remain aloof from the broader setting of social life in which people consider a problem for its ethicality in the complex setting of social, political and economic relations. Any resolution of moral crises faced in IVF thus calls for the status of women and the state of women in the society in which she is. This should be done not merely by women, any concerned feminists should come together to find out what oppression does IVF offer to women in particular and be thus connected for immorality. It is possible though that IVF and other technologies open oppressive measures for a poor husband as well for him who for his biological inabilities could not go for sexual reproduction; feminist ethics should consider this as well but in any way as Sherwin rightly thinks, not in an atomic fashion but in cooperation in society. Does this open up a door for bioethical resolution? We have to wait for our readers to find out.

Let our readers move on with their task of resolution in cooperation, but in the meantime I would like to frame a set of ethical questions in this matter to make things more interesting for them. It will be extremely interesting to find out the ways in which the set of questions here has been changed or modified by them for lively dialogues and the outcome of these dialogues. Surely, it is here I believe they would find to their wonder and much to the annoyance of Sherwin that in a model of resolution of ethical issues in IVF, the participating people after much churning about women oppression and their resolution show that theory non-cooption did not prevent them from upholding one theory, including much loved 'feminist theory'. If our readers did care for what I call "post corroboration" analysis, they are sure to find theories in function in moral resolution though none were truly theory co-opted. It is very difficult for Sherwin and other feminists, therefore, to forget the truth that knowing first about the failures or defeats of standard ethical theories and then about the success of feminist ethics does not pave way for what is known as "theory non-co-opted way" to ethical resolution. When first hand job is about theories, there is no non-cooption any further. It is better to realize the care for peoples' participation in such matters without any care on their part for theories but only for dialogue. Our ethicist, nevertheless, might find out a few interesting things later on when debate and resolution is over. Now, here is a sample set of questions for moral debate on IVF.

QUESTIONNAIRE

1. What according to you should be the aim of the bio-scientists to use reproductive technologies such as IVF?
2. Do you think that IVF is unethical because it degraded the status of naturally procreating humans who normally have families as well?

3. What is ethically good in the choice of IVF over and above the choice of adoption in case of those who can afford both? What if some people cannot afford IVF?
4. Is IVF good enough for affluent classes? If that be the case, why does satisfaction of a class justify the general goodness of IVF?
5. Is it morally just to allow biological selection of genetically rich materials for IVF?
6. Who have the moral authority for deciding participation of parties in IVF as well as for deciding sex of offspring in that process?
7. What decision-making rules would you like to see in India in case of IVF?

With this we end the ethical discussion about beginning human life. When we come to beginning mammalian life in particular, the story perhaps starts afresh with "cloning" because it is a weird biological field of beginning life of non-human animals which paves way for beginning life of humans as well. Today human cloning is not merely theoretically possible, it is practically speaking, any day affair. I would not like to enter in its details as I am more concerned in this book with ethical problems troubling a number of people in India, and cloning for sure is more of queerness among us, not posing much practical threat to Indian bio-ethicists at the present time. Still we may have a look at the problem briefly. Everyone knows Dolly the sheep; she has been made famous by Ian Wilmut and his colleagues in Roslin Institute, who cloned her on July 5, 1996, from an *adult somatic cell.* It is reported that as early as in 1960s salamander was cloned, in 1975 cloning was possible in case of adult frogs and in 1989 first piglet clone was possible. But cloning of Dolly was somewhat unique because she is not an identical clone. The technique involved transplanting the genetic material of an adult sheep into an egg from which the nucleus had been removed. The early attempts to obtain identical clones was thus overcome by obtaining genetic material of only one parent, and was, therefore, a *delayed genetic twin* of a single adult sheep. Dolly's case became an instant biological hit as it had great promises for human longevity and fertility. Keeping *human advantages* in view, therefore, Dolly, the scapegoat (!) was glorified on ethical lines because in due course we may be able to influence differentiation of somatic cells to obtain targeted cell types enabling generation of many useful tissues in human transplantation as well as Xenotransplantation. We have already seen the ethical problems in this regard but it now becomes more interesting to find that pig cloning has raised much prospect for more successful Xenotransplantation. It is not that Dolly's case has been glorified on the line of human benefits rather; mention has been made of the use of such cloning method to produce more dairy products and livestock, though with some risk that in such asexual method, a particular disease may be ever present in all clones. We know that Dolly later on developed arthritis because its adult had the problem. Yet, such animal clones raise hopes for saving and also generating endangered or rare species, which is ethical because it is *beneficial to the environment* at large. In case of humans, advantages are supposed to be greater as it raises hope for treatment of severe injuries, for bone marrow transplant, for leukemia, for degenerative diseases such as Parkinson's disease and for intractable infertility. These arguments, mostly hovering around "beneficence" hold that "The production of Dolly should not be seen as a moral threat, but rather as an exciting challenge.... In a society which is still scientifically illiterate, the onus is on researchers to explain the potential good that can be gained in the laboratory"[7].

Nevertheless, at the flip side of the coin is embossed a cry for unethicality because somatic cell nuclear transfer to create offspring raises serious question for safety, individuality, integrity of family and treating offspring, particularly humans as mere objects or commodities. Hence, cloning raised more problems for an already ethically troubled people by the act of IVF to begin life in controlled conditions. Not only this, the somatic cell nuclear transfer cloning raised value questions such as social value degradation in encouraging a queer form of eugenics, manipulation of subjects as if they were objects, hindering personal choice in procreation and bringing up child and maintaining no privacy in biological affairs. The supporters of religious ethics argue that cloning is inherently unethical in so far as it jeopardizes the nature given to animals by God. Human cloning could be taken as nothing but a gross challenge to divine act, which is however, a complete myth. Some religious people argued that environmental benefits may be too difficult to avoid. If we carefully collect the straws of 'unethicality arguments', it further amounts to that of "beneficence" because the antagonists think that cloning of humans are not of any benefit to them as they are socially and religiously damaging than helping. Greatest unethicality perhaps lies in its cruel and unethical stance towards "adoption" of the helpless orphan child and the tilt of balance of public money on huge biological expenditure of not much use because it is for a class only. Moreover, some people feel that its unethicality lies in the hopeless scientific gimmick to belie God and to naturalize everything, which is however, pointless as any natural process does not logically belie metaphysical reality. Interestingly, protagonists argue that in the fear of the death of their gods, religious people declare cloning as immoral, particularly human cloning. Still, unfazed, antagonists feel that not only human cloning, non-human animal cloning is essentially unethical because no one has the moral authority to interfere in nature's balance. Who has given the responsibility to be so sympathetic to animals to clone them? What if they were never cloned? It may well be that we saw animals as cheap things to experiment on for duplication or multiplication so that apart from much touted benefits, we eye on their nutritional value in the face of their dwindling numbers and increase in our numbers. The politics in hyped protection of animal species could be thus grossly unethical. This final point of the antagonist might raise a furore among the vegetarians and animal lovers as for the benefit of human appetite animals cannot be cloned. Among the Hindus, who think that cows are not ordinary animals, the news of hybrid cow-human embryo cell stem developed by Dr. Michael West is not welcome news either because why cows should be multiplied for human appetite is not known to them when the milk that is good enough for us is abundant in a scientific dairy upkeep.

Many antagonists hold that cloned mice apart, when we come to cloned pets such as dogs and cats for the sake of Xenotransplants, it is completely unethical because we do not have any moral right to save our lives by rearing some pets to fill up the void of one killed pet, does not solve the unethicality because non-interference in animal life is a humane and ecologically wise step than multiplying them for use. It would be interesting to know from suffering people, who, for instance, need a Xenotransplant whether or not for him or her, a pet's heart is emotionally as well as ethically acceptable. Or, more tantalizing would be to conceive of a future in which every executed human has to donate body parts to ailing people, or they clone their notorious carbon-copy or a genetically corrected more noble copy for further stay on earth – immortalized. The problem is not that immortality is not a biological issue because we should know that biologically speaking, any 'Xeroxed being' will die a natural or unnatural death, and therefore, not immortal. Hence, "immortality" cannot be an ethically glossed ideal of biology. Moreover, why should a disease free and delayed-death of human be ethically fine at the cost of other animals? What would be wrong in having 'Xeroxed humans' for his delayed-death and disease-free life? Will he be more of a psychopath or less? Are lesser psychopaths' better humans? Another trifling argument for unethicality may be that 'chimera-humans' die a thousand deaths in escaping from death because in the fear of the inevitable he causes death of several others thereby easily killing their moral sense. To end the range of arguments now, we should mention this final one from the antagonist: "The genes are in us, but we do not own the right to use or exploit them for any purpose. What is taking place is the largest game of three-card Monte in our post-modern times. As Americans and others in the world argue about the ethics of modern research, corporation's are buying up the rights to every biological process and to every life form. Capitalists' speculation has found the mother lode of all investments. What is going on is nothing less than the privatization of life itself. If scientists do succeed with stem-cell research and find a cure for diabetes, stroke, heart disease and nerve damage, the price will be exorbitant.... The potential of our own human bodies will be sold back to us – for those who can afford it – at an enormous cost"[8].

Now on the basis of the range of arguments and counter-arguments which are ethically oriented, we may further draw a list of questions for ethical debate and find for us with concerned parties, what should be done in this regard in India. Again we shall find after the post-corroboration analysis of the debate that being theory non-co-opted and not knowing anything about these arguments, we are in a good position to find our ethical replies and resolutions.

QUESTIONNAIRE

1. What according to you should be the ethically desirable goal of reproductive technologies like animal and human cloning?
2. Does cloning amount to evolutionary determinism and speciesism? If it does, is it ethically good? If it does not, what exactly does it amount to, which is also ethically good?

3. Does cloning amount to immortalizing humans? If it does, is it ethical? If it does not, what exactly is it, which is also morally good?
4. Is it ethical to have animal clones for human benefits?
5. Suggest rules for cloning of animals in view of the social, political, economic, cultural and religious factors prevailing in India.

Let us now come to the ethical debate of desirability of "killing non-human animals" for biological and medical purposes. In the former case, we include killing of non-human animals for the purposes of education, research, training and cosmetics. In the latter case, we include killing of these animals for the purposes of drug research and tests. The need for killing for "education" in biology means that all prospective zoologists and aspirants of medical course need to kill a few animals to learn something very important about animal physiology and physiological mechanisms. This is, however, legally permissible till date (at least in India) though the story may be different if there is ruthless killing in any institution. Interestingly, legally speaking, prospective physicians for their "education", particularly of human physiology need "dead human animals" or else it is not permissible. However, all dead humans cannot be dissected for education. When we come to "research, tests and training", we may conveniently skip the separation biological and medical fields because what we mean to discuss is the ethic of the killing of non-human animals for "our benefits". In this group are tests for drugs and cosmetics because they are also for "human benefits" but some drugs may be for the benefit of animals in particular. Hence, we may now concentrate on "using animals" for us for two broad reasons – education and researches. It is worth nothing here that for many of us, not all researchers on animals are for "human benefits", and not all cases of dissection amounting to death of animals are for "hùman benefits". In case of education, for proper understanding of animal physiological mechanisms, dissection is needed, which benefits humans no doubt but causes some good of animals as well. However, many others think that no education can be glorified by killing live animals (humans and non-humans) and that no research on animals benefits them. This amounts to all win-win situations for humans and total loss for animals. The tension about "killing animals" thus emanates from the question: "who wins what, when animals are killed?"

In India both the cases of killing for education and research have caused some ethical turmoil among students, teachers, scientists, medicos and common men. It has been reported that a number of Indian students have faced emotional setbacks while biological dissection sessions in classes XI and XII in our schools were in progress. Some girls could not tolerate the view of a pregnant rat when it was cut open, others could not tolerate the dissections they were purely vegetarians and some others could not tolerate the act of killing innocent creatures for learning certain things. In the late eighties, KARE (Kindness to Animals and Respect for Environment), a group of students and teachers mobilized many others to shun dissections. In 1994, the group formally requested the HRD Ministry to stop such things from school curriculum, and in 1996 they filed a petition in the Delhi High Court to stop the menace because HRD did not act properly. Their petition amounted to "right of choice" in learning about animals. In 1998 the group had much to cheer for their request was noticed by the learned court and the order for stopping dissection was made imperative in the school curriculum. Naturally the NCERT had to act appropriately drafting alternative to dissection for teaching animal physiology such as charts and 3-D images. Yet, many private schools continued with dissection. The matter gained some back-up from the Prevention of Cruelty to Animals Act of 1960 which states the desirability of avoiding dissection of animals for teaching. KARE finds support from many people, even the biologists and physicians. Dr. Jerry Vlasak, MD, of American Board of Surgery told in 1998 in a seminar in Kolkata that "The best way to learn about human anatomy is by studying humans, not animals"[9]. He said that dissection on animals is merely a matter of convenience rather than being *humane*. The question of ethicality thus creeps in the debate.

When we come to the field of research on animals, we have more interesting clashes between scientists and supporters of animal care. An interesting list of such clash was provided in the daily, *The Times of India* of March 25, 2002. The Committee for the Purpose and Supervision of Experiments of Animals under the Union ministry of Social Justice and Empowerment and the Laboratory of Animal Sciences, Hyderabad stopped the Indian Institute of Science, Bangalore and All India Institute of Medical Sciences, New Delhi from research on monkeys. The Institute for Research in Reproduction, Mumbai was not allowed to proceed by the CPCSEA for its project on large animals. The LV Prasad Institute for Eye in Hyderabad was not allowed by the CPCSEA to experiment on eyes of animals for the treatment of glaucoma and cataract. AIIMS also got a setback on vaccine research when it was prevented from using monkeys. The researchers complain that the CPCSEA in the name of animal rights forgot that the students of post-graduation are heckled by *ethics committees* to clear research projects. The CPCSEA on the other hand reported that every year in India more than 50 lakh animals which include rats, snakes, frogs, monkeys, horses and buffaloes are being experimented upon by various research laboratories across the country. In these ultramodern labs, animals live in a dingy condition, mostly ill treated and malnourished. Interestingly the Government of India allowed exporting some 20 lakh monkeys in 1978 for nuclear researches which was protested by animal rights people, which went in vain but since then use of animals in India increased threefold. This is not only due to lackadaisical approach of the Indian government from time to time but owing to expansion of multinational drug companies and research labs who could comfortably research on animals without much hoopla. These labs go on abusing animals in experiments and these experiments are oft repeated. Astounding figure of animals killed in educational institutions (22 lakhs per year) is worth considering. The gruesome killing of animals in India in the modern labs are not merely for saving life of humans, there are a number of cosmetic tests on animals which cannot be life-saving by any extension of the term. Most cosmetic users however are unaware of the number of tests on animals being conducted before marketing these costly things. Reportedly, shampoo concentrate for instance, is tested on rabbit's eyes; monkeys are fed with lipsticks, hair dyes and talcum powder for test of toxicity. Civets are beaten up for secretion of musk in their pouch. The Association of Beauty without Cruelty tries to control manufacturers in the abuse of animals but least care is shown towards them. Even the Bureau of Indian Standards in 1997 thought that tests on animals were not necessary but it added to state that when deemed necessary for safety, tests may be conducted. Most of these tests are age-old, very rustic so to say, and those who survive it become trash, to be killed later on. It is painful to listen that the Draize test of 1937 for blinding monkeys for cosmetics is still in practice.

Now the antagonists and protagonists with regard to the ethic of tests and research on animals have interesting arguments. We have seen in an earlier discussion that we view non-human animals in distinct ways in comparison to the value of humans; for instance, we value non-human animals for their existence on earth for maximization of our good. Hence, some animal existence on earth may be abruptly ended. However, ending human existence for maximization of human good is not a welcome idea in normal cases; in abnormal cases like wars, maximization of good of some humans may be possible by killing some humans but that is "abnormal". Yet, if some of us believe that killing some non-human animals for human good is not a good idea, then one hopefully considers these non-human animals as "persons", which is, however, extremely unacceptable "literally". This is so because our conception about "human persons" is based on so-called "intrinsic properties" of which non-biological ones are most striking. Some people consider "consciousness" as the crucial property (and strangely non-biological) whereas others think that "intentions" and "morally chosen actions for goodness and rightness" are crucial. It is not difficult to find out people who think that "religiosity" is the most crucial property. If we skip biological criteria such as nature of chromosomes (this we have already discussed), the above "intrinsic-to-human properties" are either redundant or misconceived. It is a misconception, because monkeys and gorillas differ from humans in so far as they have lower degree of consciousness. A little care will enable us to believe that the categories of "intentional moral choice and action" and "religiosity" are meaningful for humans because that distinguishes one type of human being from other human beings but not applicable in any sense to non-human animals. It is essentially foolish to say that as some animals like gorillas are not religious, they are not *like* human beings in many other ways. Hence, the above criteria are redundant. In a *figurative* way to use "persons" for *some* non-human animals, what is conceived is the sense of "as valuable a being in nature as humans are" for several biological and evolutionary, ecological and economic reasons. Hence, one may hold as Peter Singer that "It sounds odd to call an animal a person. This oddness may be no more than a symptom of our habit of keeping our own species sharply separated from others. In any case, we can avoid the linguistic oddness by rephrasing the question in accordance with our definition of 'person'"[10]. He further holds that "If human life does have special value, it has it in so far as most human beings are persons. But if some non-human animals are persons too, there must be the same value in the lives of those animals"[11]. In that case, these valuable creatures like chimpanzees, gorillas etc. *should not* be killed for maximizing human good. Speciesism that champions greater value of humans may be emotive but the one championing only value of humans and the use of non-humans as means to human good must be *unethical* or *ethically undesirable*. It is interesting to notice that though much tear is shed for a human turned to a vegetative condition by losing its holy "consciousness" is in no case comparable to the value of a gorilla which is keeping fit, and for that reason, its killing for humans cannot be ethical either. Or, if it be good, shedding tear for our poor vegetative kin and fellow men is without any sense, they may be killed happily. Thus a human being who has lost the status of a "person" though not better than a gorilla who is still having biological *value* does not stand termination of life as the gorilla does not. Strangely, our legal system in most civil states does not recognize these animals as "persons" and are not as emphatic in either deterrence or retribution as they are when even vegetative humans are withdrawn from a life sustaining system without consent or when they are simply killed as Dr. Death (Kevorkian) does. Why should intentional killing of chimpanzees be legally approached in a lax fashion? Certainly, they are not "person" as we are. It is due to this that a number of these poor creatures are exported from their African resorts to hi-tech multinational labs to be tested and subsequently killed for human well-being. This is essentially unethical as there is gross violation of rights and dignity of some valuable non-human lives which are not caressed and cared as our pets, which we grudgingly or gladly take as "persons". It is extremely morally wrong, therefore, to kill any animal without judging for its value as a person and treating them as mere means for our good. The arguments of the antagonists of killing animals have thus taken a good start.

When we come to the justification of taking life of some animals for human benefits though these animals have very low or meager consciousness, the antagonist have something more to say. They argue that any use of animal irrespective of their levels of consciousness, for our good, is ethically unjustifiable. Hence, it is not only in case of chimpanzees and gorillas, rather when we consume fishes, chickens and a number of birds to meet our protein demands, such killings are equally unethical. It is not very difficult to imagine that among these animals, particularly some birds, a close relationship lasting for a long time between male and female could be seen. In that case, taking life of one member causes some irreparable suffering to the other member, which can be realized, if not computed because what degree of wailing amounts to unbearable animal pain is not known to us in any objective way. Similarly, being humans (if we really are), we have some sense of pain and loss in taking life, which is true for any life being taken on earth. Why then animal life of any form would not eke out a small sense of pain in us is not understandable. Enjoying or causing or being a party to infliction of pain on other living beings who could neither appropriately stand for self-defence nor claim rights, is ethically wrong. The ethical wrongness is not merely due to killing rather killing made glorious for human good. Why should human good so heavily depend merely on other selves? Why should it be so glorious? Is it true that without consuming and using these animals our good is not possible? The antagonists also argue against the view that though humans kill animals for consuming meat in particular, they are also benevolent in the creation and nurturing of a lot of animals, whose number might outwit the number of those killed. The antagonists hold that any life on earth in itself is not replaceable by virtue of creation and rearing of animals because the way the animal farms treat these animals is in reality burdensome for their life. The natural right of animals to get some "pleasure", whatever "gross" that may be from our perception, is certainly not replaceable. Interesting is to know whether or not protagonists would kill their pet dogs when they grow older and lose their desired beauty and replace them with another cute dog? And whether or not they would replace their own children when they grow up to replace them by their clones? Further, who on earth has given us the noble duty to create animals for our population which needs to be fatter. What if we did not get fatter eating meat though unlike animals, we had little or no wisdom to check our population? Our population has still on hand land to cultivate food to feed than create animals for food. In case of arid and cold zones, the possibility of cultivation may be ruled out, but in the present world we do not live in distant, isolated villages that have no access to basic food like rice, wheat, maize and so on. Hence, killing animals for eating meat is unjustifiable on the ethical ground of maximizing human good. Rather, to consider human and non-human lives as equally valuable is ethically justifiable as that does more good in the world on the whole. If we now compare a human being who has no aspiration for life, does not procreate and hopefully is in pain but is not able to aspire longer life or a healthier life in the future, with the animal life of a healthy, procreating, happy gorilla then certainly we harm them while reducing their happiness on earth on the whole for our happiness. Even if such animals are replaceable by virtue of cloning or artificial procreation, we surely fail to replace the "happiness" of the living beings killed on earth, and if we fail to contribute in that fashion, we have no moral authority to kill them.

At the flip side of the coin is, however, mild protagonist argument to kill those animals who are not as self-conscious as many animals like chimpanzees and gorillas. Peter Singer draws such conclusion in his work *Practical Ethics* after rejecting the ethical validity of killing any animal on earth on some utilitarian grounds, he thinks that a utilitarian might still successfully argue as based on the basic difference between self-conscious and not so self-conscious animals that the latter beings have a valuable life, which has its biological worth, is happy enough, contributes to happiness in the world, procreates but most importantly it fails to *urge for a healthy life in future*, and, therefore, does not strive to lead a healthy life. In this sense, for them life and death does not make much sense as it does for humans and non-human self-conscious animals. Hence, proper ways to use them and to replace them may be no less utilitarian. He says: "This means that in some circumstances when animals lead pleasant lives, are killed painlessly, their deaths do not cause suffering to other animals, and the killing of one animal makes possible its replacement by another who would not otherwise have lived, the killing of non-self conscious animals may not be wrong".[12] It appears that Singer has been finally compelled to accept killing of birds who are supposedly not self-conscious on the main utilitarian consideration that in cases of human existence depending only on such animals we would ethically justify killing ducks but not gorillas. This would be comparable to a tiger killing deer for its bare existence because it cannot feed on grass and does not prefer eating rats. It is thus natural for people like Singer or others who live in places where it is not difficult to imagine a state of life without plenty vegetables and corns, killing is but natural. Moreover, such killings being not passionate and ruthless, easily balances the existence of the species by back up procreation, natural and artificial. This may be true in case of research as well, particularly when humans are not available for it for bare existence, when mice, rats and lower beings may be *used* for greater good.

The protagonists of killing some animals at least thus make the debate more interesting. However, we have still not come across the cases of killing animals as justified not for bare existence, but for different tests for the benefit of humans. What would protagonists say in such cases? In this case the protagonists generally perform a negative task first. They first *refute* that non-human animals, self-conscious or not so, do not enjoy "rights". Further, they argue that they do not enjoy any right to not to be used and subsequently killed by humans for greater human good as well as good of the animal health and procreation. Hence, animals need to be killed if necessary in different tests and researches. Most expectedly, therefore, the antagonists' base their arguments on animals enjoying rights such as not to be killed in tests and researches. Naturally we have to consider the crucial question of rights of animals. It will be very interesting here to consider the arguments of the antagonist Tom Regan, and the protagonist Carl Cohen. However, there are many more worth considering essays, which we need not take at this place for all practical purposes. Tom Regan thinks that those who imagine that animals have rights rejects the so-called "human and humane benefits" of use of animals such as rats because that amounts to deliberate "harm", which cannot be allowed as animals enjoy the *right to be unharmed by humans* as they are not valuable merely as "receptacle" or "means" for human good. Excluding this sense of "rights" of animals, Regan clarifies that these creatures enjoy the *rights of not to be reduced to "objects of use", "fulfilling the human aspirations", "something which helps in proving a hypothesis", "something that helps in constructing a new insight"* and *"something beneficial to others"*. In other words, rats and animals like these do have right to live a life free of intentionally inflicted pain by humans. They are not valuable because humans perceive them as such, that is, having some "use-value", where "use" is only "human-use". Further, extension of what has been said above amounts to the truism that animals have right to pose a mute challenge at least to prevent the practice of tests and researches on them for the interests of other parties. In this way they also challenge the perception that animals are renewable resources. Hence, they enjoy the right of not to be treated as bare commodities in nature which needs to be killed and created at human wish. This amounts to the view that rights of animals are based on "intrinsic value" of their being in nature and their contributions to the biotic-community, which certainly humans tend to forget because they always prefer to be the Pied Piper ready to kill rats at any cost. If this be the case, rights of animals are tantamount to a mute claim to *respect* their *autonomy* and their value so that "institutionalizing" them as not something to be "respected for value" is stopped. Regan says, therefore, that "Scientific research, when it involves routinely harming animals in the name of possible "human and humane benefits", violates this requirement of respectful treatment. Animals are not to be treated as mere receptacles or as renewable resources. This practice of scientific research on animals violate their rights. Thus it ought to cease, according to the rights view".[13] It amounts to say that animal rights call for not using animals in any case, that is, it is not a good excuse to say that only after sincere efforts to find alternatives for researches, animals were chosen. Hence, animals cannot be used as the only alternative or as the last resort. Similarly, animal rights amount to rejection of the so-called careful or judicious use of animals in research, but after all our efforts if they had to die, they should die. This is so because the inherent value of animals remains constant whether or not they are ruthlessly or are judiciously used. Use is after all "use", and for Regan, "The best we can do in terms of not using animals is not to use them"[14]. Clearly, the unethicality of killing animals in scientific researches is based on human conception of animals as *mere means* to their own good.

Regan clarifies that the conception of animal rights enables us to realize the ethicality of those uses of animals in research which ultimately help scientists to find out *remedies* for the sick individuals, both human and non-human. Here is a twist of pen by Regan. He now clarifies that "any non-use of animals in research" should not extend to non-use in the benefit of animals themselves or other the sick animals. Equally true is that sick human animals stand a just claim for healthier life and should be thus treated adequately. Clearly, Regan now speaks of some unavoidable *use* of animals which is human and humane not because it helps animals as well but it helps the *neediest individuals*. Animal rights thus amount to declare the *unethicality* of animals in researches injudicious and ruthless, that is, in researches not of any use to the "sick individuals". Animal rights for Regan are thus an ethical movement for it tries to stop the intentional menace on lab animals. However, in case of animal benefits, that is, to help the sick ones, any study and research needs to be conducted in labs and not in the jungles perhaps, which is also a well deliberated act. How will Regan answer this? Better asked, why should we not pick some human individuals first for tests and studies for benefit of animals in a cozy atmosphere rather than animals put in cages? Perhaps Regan has in mind "stacking", "stocking" and "sticking" animals in lab conditions for avoidance of all that would be "humane". Perhaps he thinks that choice of humans than animals is unethical because we are too few and they are too many. But in the latter case the Indian and the Chinese should be very good volunteers through consent. Or, are they not? May be, animals are more easily "replaced" than humans and the process may be "cost effective" as well. If that be the case, humans are still in an all win-win position. But let us not be complaining; let us try to understand Regan in a better way.

Regan further says that animal rights are not either an unscientific or an anti-scientific standpoint because it does not declare a blanket ban on animal research on ethical basis. Equally true is that it does not gloss humane use of animals in research by providing AC labs, clean conditions, good food, anesthetized experiments and post-operative care because in any case these things cannot minimize harm, pain and suffering of animals. This being the case, we are naturally turned to rely on human volunteers and not the sick individuals, but that has its own problems of unethicality. In the face of this embarrassing situation Regan holds that "If non-animal alternatives are available, they should be used; if they are not available, they should be sought. That is the moral challenge to research, given the rights view, and it is those scientists who protest that this cannot be done in advance of the scientific commitment to try—not those who call for exploration, who exhibit a lack of commitment to, and belief in the scientific enterprise, who are, that is, anti-scientific at the deepest level"[15]. What we got from this is that the ethicality of not killing animals stands a solid ground if and only if proper *alternatives* are found in scientific research because Regan and all others like us are worried about good life and not premature death and unnecessary suffering for the animals. It is extremely bad on the part of the scientists, therefore, to put down their heads and drop shoulders before the fight for finding humane alternatives is not over. But if there is no way out, human volunteers and animals both should be *used* for the general biological welfare of animals. Still I must remind that non-human animals will never consent for all this; we need to seek such consent too from our conscience and from the conscientious scientific and non-scientific fraternity. Given these ethical arguments and the sense of protection of rights of animals, it is difficult to declare it as anti-human or anti-scientific or anti-animal. It is welcome, though emotionally intolerable at times to accept the truth that whenever inhuman treatment of animals is stopped, it would cause some retardation in scientific ventures leading to cure of diseases but that is fine because whenever we faced insoluble threats to our life, we stood up, fought and overcame the threats. What Regan finally holds about this matter is against all forms of utilitarian arguments, some of which Peter Singer trashed (the receptacle theory in particular) and some which he did not, that is, his own theory, though with some modification and partial acceptance. Regan would have no hesitation is *using human and non-human animals* with *consent* in *decent atmosphere* in scientific researches for *bare existence* of humans as well as non-humans (this Singer overlooked). Did Regan sidestep utilitarianism or all forms of consequentialism in this way? Perhaps no, because he does accept the truth that saving life for existential good on the whole is ethically good. Readers of Mill's *Utilitarianism* realize that utilitarian consequentialism is not blind to animal-good. In fact, *biological welfarism* (about which we knew in the previous ethical debate), does happily accept Regan and Singer with some qualification.

Carl Cohen in his essay, *"Do Animals Have Rights?"*[16] asks to consider this question seriously because it decides the ethicality of protecting the rights of animals at great costs if needed. Cohen, like many others, such as, Joel Feinberg defines "rights" in terms of "claim rights" because that is the basic sense of the term which as if carrying a "legal" flavour ought to be protected at some cost but it is also important to remember that such "claims" are made by "moral agents" under "principles that govern both the claimant and the target of the claim"[17]. This does not rule out one possibility. I must mention that animals do not utter any claim language but we all do but that does not prove that only utterer of the language have such claim. Even if sane people utter claims for animals or rights so to say, would be as good as *having* them for the animals. Hence, the stress on "moral agents" must be carefully scrutinized as we proceed with the views of Cohen. Cohen warns us that if some people think that though animals have rights such as not to be ruthlessly experimented and killed, they do not surpass *our* rights any way. This is a poor argument thinks Cohen because the argument has not even a shaky premise of why human claims are overriding; rather, it shows that if we have rights which should be protected, then their rights should be protected as well. Cohen argues that vaccines for killer diseases of epidemic proportions like polio is available to us today because our scientists successfully developed them and tested on mice for guarantee and safety. He says, this is done "because there is no other way" and that "we will never have such vaccines". We all expect that Cohen must have thought carefully as Regan did in terms of our best way to prevent human callousness in scientific researches, that is, to make no sincere effort to avoid use of animals. Now, if this be the case, Regan and others would hardly object that mice should be saved any way even if people died of polio or whatever. But things are not as simple as Cohen hits the crux of the issue by refuting the idea of animals having claim rights to not to be killed in medical research. Hence, even if Cohen sounds like Regan in justifying the necessary use of mice in research, the basis of coming to this conclusion is different. Cohen bases it on animals having no claim rights to not to be killed, to which Regan does not agree. Moreover, as we shall see that Cohen's conclusion may not be the same as Regan because Cohen may be far more liberal in the use of mice in research than Regan. Cohen's concern in this regard is that important medical researches essentially depend on the use of mice and other animals, which cannot and should not stop because in doing so using animals, big or small for our diet has to be stopped. Further, any technological aid such as computer simulations for biomedical researches in place of live animals could be bogus. Naturally, either we stop investigations and prepare to die or we are saved if mice die. Hence, Cohen thinks that to stop this way of thinking he should explain "why animals cannot possess claim rights" and why taking their life for good reasons is good itself.

Cohen thinks that humans are obliged to animals in many ways but that does not logically entail that animals have a claim that humans remain obliged to them by not using them for good reasons. In fact, all rights entail obligations but not all obligations entail rights. Surely, I am obliged to my teachers for what they have taught to me but my teachers cannot claim that they enjoy the right that I will send them a complementary copy of this book. Though when I was their student, my right to get information from them entailed that there is at least someone who is obliged to give me the necessary information for which I paid. Thus we are not legally or morally bound to not to kill the mice even if we are obliged to hundreds of them who died for us. It is crucial to remember, therefore, that even if animals have tremendous value in biotic community, even if we are really obliged to them, we sued to kill some of them for a greater biological good than killing humans to whom perhaps we are not obliged in any way. The queer reason is owing to the fact that even the most ungrateful and non-obliged people enjoy certain claim rights such as not to be killed, which tragically non-moral beings like mice do not enjoy. Yet, there is no reason to think that, therefore, humans suddenly enjoy the right to kill as many mice as they wish, to treat them with all disregard and to torture them because humans qua humans have no moral authority to behave in an awkward inhuman way such as to inflict pain at their will for nothing. Hence, humans cannot become insensitive creatures even if animals enjoy no rights. Cohen thus brings out the truth that as the conception of "rights" is human, it is not true in case of animals. It is a confusion, therefore, to extend rights to animals but it is logically perfect to use and to subsequently kill some animals for greater cause. This enables us to use animals in medical research in a more noble way. Cohen puts it in these words: "When using animals in our research, therefore, we ought to indeed be humane – but we can never violate the rights of those animals because to be blunt, they have none. Rights do not apply to them"[18]. This further enables us to say that in killing animals in medical research we have committed no crime but in deliberately killing thousands of chickens in a poultry farm and to kill a notoriously ungrateful man is certainly a crime. The latter is the case because in both the instances of killing chickens and ungrateful man, we are either violating the claim right of hundreds of people who depended on the poultry farm products for food at some cost or we are violating the claim right of the person to live unharmed life though by nature he is ungrateful. This may be now easily contrasted with killing thousands of poultry chickens during SARS epidemic and slaughter hundreds of cows when foot and mouth disease spreads. Such killings were essential as thousand of animals, including humans would have died otherwise. I fear that the most revered animals in different parts of the world have to be killed in such cases, and the argument to not to consume these animals, is ethically good, is childish, for we feed or not, the epidemic does not spare us, they attack through contacts and contaminations. Interestingly, the argument that if no body fed on chickens, there would be no SARS epidemic and thus chickens need not be killed, is not a safe argument either because in that way to stop many diseases we have to quit eating and drinking, which will further cause malnutrition – another disease. More interesting is to notice that our most sincere efforts to find a SARS vaccine will be ever active on earth to save our and chickens' lives if and only if some of them die in the process of medical tests for effectiveness of the vaccine on them.

Cohen tries to refute Regan's (and many others') popular conception that animals, like humans have inherent value, that is, value not merely as means to the maximization of good of others rather, value as such. This is crucial in our understanding of why ruthless killing of animals, even smaller ones by humans is so unethical because every petty (!) animal lives a unique life in the biotic community, they are all crucial in that community's structure, balance and harmony, and we do not have any legal and moral right to kill them for fun or for sale in large numbers. This is especially true of the endangered or near extinct species. Again we find here that apart from inhuman and immoral approaches, it is our claim right that all of us (including animals) need to live at a place where biological balance is not rampaged. However, Cohen says that when Regan draws another sense of "inherent value" of animals for their non-killing, it is unacceptable to him. Regan conceives of animals and humans both having "inherent value" in the sense of "moral autonomy" as well as "subject-of-a-life", which is unacceptable to Cohen for its ambiguity and category confusion. Animals, as they have no claim rights, does not have "moral" autonomy either because that is true of humans and none of the other beings. What "subject-of-a-life" is, is more unclear. Cohen thinks that Regan plays on the vague use of the notion "inherent value" in each case in this regard and perhaps slips to what he calls, the *fallacy of equivocation*, that is, wrong use of words or in premises of arguments. Hence, if animals have inherent value as members of biotic community they have no inherent value to be treated as moral agents enjoying claim right to not to be killed in medical researches. Rather, they should be used and if needed killed for discoveries in saving lives of humans as well as animals (but strangely), this is not true of human subjects for experiments because for Cohen the category of rights, including moral rights is applicable only in case of human beings, and medical science aims at human good but not by taking their lives if needed. But why moral agents as we surely are having several rights and reasons are not subject to researches? To be sure, voluntary human subjects are always better subjects practically speaking than mice for here we do not depend on any biological deduction rather direct experience involving human body. Why should human rights be not extended to morally acting for a benevolent cause such as medical research? Does rights logically entail that humans need not and should not give life (and for that matter be killed by someone) if need for humanity at large? It is also interesting to notice that there can be no logical entailment between exclusive claim rights of humans for non-killing of other humans and themselves for medical research and killing. Suppose a street-dog is truly not a moral agent and truly do not have claim right such as not to be taken for polio vaccine then from these does it logically follow that only they need to be killed? Suppose computer simulated mechanisms are bogus in medical research and teaching, does it further logically follow that we are left with dogs and cats for medical research? One may ask, who then need to be killed if not cats and dogs taking it to be true that for medical research a living being is needed (preferably mammals)? The answer needs another false question to be asked because the one asked here is "false" in nature because it suggested that cats and dogs are to be killed in research and none else; the question is: what if human volunteers consent to such research? Does moral beings having claim rights for unharmed life be not a party to benevolent act like this one?

Readers have noticed by this time that there is much tension among varieties of utilitarian thinkers and the non-utilitarian thinkers regarding this matter, but strangely, both are happy to conclude that any biological good done to animals as such, which includes humans as well in medical research is ethically good, and for this abuse of any animal in the labs is ethically wrong. Moreover, none is courageous to say that death is a natural phenomenon in nature for all beings, so let it come in due course even premature and in epidemic proportions without any medical intervention. The advanced psychopaths who would have preferred this option are not the ones we have discussed here and if there are some more burdening the world till date or in future, let us ignore their views but do not ignore them as persons for they need treatment – they are sick. I know that even this would cause ethical furore, but let it be like that for that stimulates my cause of dialogue. Another point is that intentional "abuse" of animals *in the name of* biological research is not restricted to the poor upkeep and dealing with the animals, rather it includes cosmetic and toiletry tortures on animals. Our debates would not accept that having rights or no rights do not hinder in declaring the unethicality of these tortures on animals. However such declaration further emanates from *two perceptions*: one is human perception of animals as having no rights but some values to be cared for and the other is human perception of animals as having some rights and some values to be cared for. In any case, it is *we*, who look at animals in different ways regarding their intrinsic and extrinsic values, it is *we*, who talk ethically about them, it is *we* who talk legally about them and it is *we* who do *not* prefer talking ethically and legally about them. There is a lot of relativism, therefore, which cannot be resolved if we do not participate in a dialogue now. Here is the questionnaire (which you may modify, if needed), to have an ethical dialogue aimed at resolution of the issue.

QUESTIONNAIRE

1. What is your perception about the relationship among man and other members of the animal kingdom?
2. Do you think that the animals in any way are valuable? Do you think that using animals in medical research and teaching is to disregard the value of animals?
3. Keeping in mind the truth that only humans can consent to medical researchers and tests leading to death in some cases, is it ethically good to go for such researches with consenting humans but not animals?
4. Keeping the same thing in mind, what would be your ethical opinion regarding use of humans and animals in furtherance of medical teaching and biological knowledge of beings?
5. Do you think that the consented use of homeopathic drugs and uninformed tests for placebo effects on humans are ethically desirable?
6. Should we use animals as well as humans for tests of cosmetic and toiletries? If yes, what is the judicious use, and if no, why should we not do so even if done judiciously?
7. Who should be accountable to conduct medical researches using humans and animals? What decision-making rules do you suggest in this regard?

After considering the value-laden issues in killing animals in biomedicine, we come to more delicate issue of taking life of humans in biomedicine. As I have already mentioned, I would like to stress more on the issue of ethic of abortion of human fetus through medical intervention and relatively less on the ethic of euthanasia in the way I have done in this chapter that is, raising the value-laden questions, the ethical tension and presenting a questionnaire for dialogue and decision-making. Let us come to the issue of *abortion* now. It is important at the outset to remember that like every other value-laden issue, abortion is a case to be considered in the unique social context where it is practiced. As such we should have special care for the Indian social context where it is practiced. Abortion in India has become a matter of great concern not in the context of the social tension owing to *religious animosity*, as it is mainly in Europe and America where people of certain faith quarrel among themselves about its ethical value and disvalue, rather, in the context of the social tension owing to *sex imbalance* in human population in India, that is, an imbalance in sex ratio of male and female population. The terrible state of affair, a kind of a slippery slope through which the female population did not only slide into a limbo, their social, political and economic standards have slipped to almost a point of no-return. By the year 2004 in the Northern states and in the Hindi Heartland, in particular, women-folk have been marginalized for existence, subsistence and growth. It is a pity to find that in some Indian states the number of females has come down below 800 marks in comparison to the male population. And it is a matter of worry for all sane and sexually normal human in India that the nation must be either crazily heading towards massive sainthood or polyandry or perversion of women. In any case the time has come to think and act about this menace. One interesting aspect of the falling number of females and their falling social status is rampant abortions all over India by quacks, untrained midwives and nurses, that is, the act is either medical intervention, scientifically done or it is rudimentary art, most unscientifically done. If one goes deeper to find the reasons, they are very complex because queer interplay of social and economic reasons makes things like that. No less important are the overwhelming dogmas, beliefs and obsessions about women. It is not our task to analyze these things; we are rather more interested in knowing about the ethical justification or rejection of abortion done medically and extra-medically. What is worrying about these "extra-medical" ways of abortion is that they are direct threat to life and of course to the fetus or potent life though that is a debat issue. In any way, whether or not fetuses are living beings, the carrier of the same is living and cannot die with the fetus at the hand of some quacks (or even doctors) for filthy reasons. Further, what is worrying about "medical abortion" by trained people is that they too have many times filthy grounds to terminate "female fetus" and even fetuses of any sex. When I speak of these "filthy grounds", I mean unethical or undesirable grounds, to which many people disagree or even if they agree they think that their overwhelming stronger reasons to abort outweighs the "filth", and, therefore, ethical. These people resort to enlist a number of reasons why fetuses must be aborted for human good, which one cannot overlook. We have to go through these ethical justifications and disagreements about non-abortion.

If we think carefully, "extra-medical" abortion by quacks (not to be confused with abortion by trained midwives and nurses at remote places or villages), does not make a valid case for ethical scrutiny because professionally, theoretically and legally abortion without scientific knowledge and procedures is not abortion at all, even if it is consented because the consent and needs apart, persons without proper knowledge and expertise abort as a matter of undue privilege they have acquired in the society and it is a chance that they succeed in killing one and saving other. We take it for granted that when someone does not legally and scientifically enjoy the status of aborting fetuses from human body is not an aborting expert or a professional but a self declared expert "killer". And not knowing the prevalent legal system or by overlooking it if someone does something grave with human body, ethicality will come next, legality will come first to punish or debar him from the act unless there are some loopholes in the system itself which calls for a revaluation and rejoinder. Hence, we are here not concerned with non-professionals rather we are concerned with professionals in the health care system who under law carry on termination of fetuses from female body preventing prospective healthy or unhealthy beings to come into existence. This is our concern because we find here sharp disagreements about the act itself which people think should not be.practiced even if law permits under certain limitations to do, and for that matter the overreaching law needs some correction as well. Now if we succeed in arguing that legally permissible act of abortion is itself unethical, the legality of the matter is relegated to a secondary affair because more overriding is the ethical scrutiny of both the act and the law which permits it. However, this is not true of "extra-medical" termination because in this case law remains overriding, not secondary in the face of moral scrutiny because morality kept in abeyance in such cases, legality is sufficient to stop *non-pragmatic*, *inhuman*, *chauvinistic*, *wishful* and *whimsical* acts. Hence, "extra-medical" abortion remains a *legally unjustifiable* issue. This is true in case of those abortions conducted by quacks which on medial inquiry were found to be too good for the woman aborted because in any case, we should not allow quacks to assume important professional role of a scientist for any stray good reason. If this is allowed, rampant malpractice spreads in health care and with it the death rates go up. However, this should be never confused with "bare foot doctors" in health care because such people as well as trained village midwives and nurses receive scientific training, they thus assume the responsibilities of *sub-professionals* (see the Primer, Vol.1) and thus enjoy legal advantage to abort, if needed. In their case, as in the case of the physicians, abortion still is a matter of ethical inquiry because legality apart, certain questions of "desirability" still need to be resolved. Let us, therefore, take it for guaranteed that we should speak about the *ethic of medical termination of pregnancy* or the *ethic of abortion* as we briefly (sometimes confusingly), call it. It is also worth noting here that we are also not worried about "spontaneous abortion" or "miscarriages" here because such physical maladies do not stand for reasonable moral debate. We are thus speaking about the *ethic of medically induced abortion*. However, we are not sure that all "medically induced abortions" are consented, that is, with the consent of the aborted woman *without any force or pressure*. In any case, we shall speak about the ethical question about "induced abortion".

Any ethical discussion about induced abortion has to keep in mind that though the controversy is about ending something growing within human females, the status of "something" is very important because if a lump is taken out of our body we do not mind much but if it is potent life, we do mind. There is a habit among the "pro" and the "con" proponents of the ethic of abortion that they use certain biological notions related to abortion differently, causing different shades of emotive exhortations about the matter. The *con-people* (who disfavour abortion), or, whom we call *pro-life people* prefer to give unique meaning and status to any state of pregnancy or gestation. For them, whether it is zygote or embryo or fetus or child, they may be referred to as states of "life" or "potent life". In this sense, "child" for them is not post-fetus state of pregnancy; any state of pregnancy from shortly after conception onward for them is a state of "life". Hence, any state where there in induced abortion, it is abortion of life in a well thought out way, which is thus "taking life" of a human by another human. There is a distinct "emotional" jerk in *pro-life* view because nobody likes his or her "child" to be aborted by any means and by any person. But, the pro view (for they favour abortion), or, whom we call pro-abortionists, are not moved by those bogus things because for them (though they are not "anti-life"), it is crucial to distinguish between stages of gestation to find out when, why and by which methods the stage may be aborted safely without much emotional honcho, and by any imagination what they call "child", the post-fetus stage (eighth week until birth), does not make a good cause for abortion. This is so because at very later stages, say at the stage of viability (twenty-sixth to twenty-eighth week), the abortion is risky, emotively and ethically unacceptable as well. It is interesting to notice however that at the sixteenth week of pregnancy it is possible to conduct amniocentesis and other investigations for tests of sex and abnormalities, and if needed, abortion may be necessary at times or is done in compulsion or consent but at that stage too, things may not be so easy and safe either. But the crux of the debate between the "pro" and the "con" views is that whether or not at any stage of gestation abortion is ethical. Hence, it is a misconception to think that for the "con" view only post-investigation information period's abortion is opposed for unethicality. (Please notice that this is "pro-life view" and both "pro" terms need not be confused because for me, "pro view" is favourable to abortion view but not "con-life view"). Interestingly, for "pro" view, pre and post-investigation information period for sexual and deformities may be ethically deemed to be just for abortion owing to several reasons. Keeping these things in minds, we can say that any state of gestation, that is, confirmed conception to viability stands out for a "pro" and "con" debate for abortion. This is nicely summed up by Daniel Callahan's notion of "conceptus" or "that which is conceived"[19], which carefully sidesteps all emotiveness in ethical debate. It is now a matter to find out why induced abortion is ethically good or bad when it comes to abort "conceptus". This is a good way to discuss the matter because for people like me who as corroborators want to remain non-committal before ethical debates should choose "conceptus" for abortion debate because it sidesteps the several technical aspects of conception. The basic value-laden problem in abortion is whether or not we have any moral authority to medically intervene in ending life, if for sure what we end is truly "life". The "surety" element in taking "life" is extremely important, therefore, because indirectly we assume that if something is testimony to "life", we need to terminate it if that is for the greater benefit of the carrier of the stuff. Then we have the biological squabble: When does human life begin? The weird realm of life puts several biological jargons for us to decide. When conceptus is bearer of life, is a matter of debate till date. Some people say that biology saved philosophy (when linguistic philosophy nearly killed it perhaps), but we find that the clarification of the concept of "life" may save us from an endless ethical impasse. Now, I have no task to take up this analysis here as that is not my project but I will surely tell my readers how different opinions regarding the sense of "life" and its "beginning" in human is related to its "taking" or "killing" or "ending". For a starter, the *pro-abortion view* of the controversy whether or not conceptus is bearer of life does not hinder abortion because if abortion is a necessity, it is *good* to abort it provided the carrier (mother), is right and free in allowing aborting. For the "con-view" (anti-abortion view), it is either ethically *bad* to abort conceptus at any stage whatever may be the rights and freedom of its carrier or it is ethically *bad* to abort the same unless it is medically urgent to do so for saving the life of the carrier and/or the prospective child. It is reasonable to imagine that though both views care for "life", none is truly "con-life" (as biologists cannot be so when mentally sound). However, one view gives great importance to the *pragmatic* aspect of the science and the female human who is the carrier of conceptus, whereas the other view gives more value to the conceptus for *extra-pragmatic* reasons. I use "extra pragmatic" to clarify that for many "con" supporters though rights and freedom of carrying women are glossed ideas, to put their and their child's life at risk is not. Hence, though pragmatics is one aspect of abortion, we have something "extra" for rejoinder, that is, the *right and good* of the conceptus which cannot suffer death when it has neither chosen life nor the end of it. Similarly, among the "pro" thinkers, though pragmatics of abortion is of great value, they are careful in debating whether or not what they abort is really "living" because when truly that term may be affixed, it is medically or pragmatically dangerous to abort. Hence, for them monitoring the stages fit for abortion is more important because they are doubly respectful for life. Clearly, the "pro" view is "pro" always to *early abortion* and not at the stage of "viability". But the "con" speakers think that though more and more you move in the scale of "viability", the more prone you are to invite danger, nevertheless even at "early stages", you invite the danger of being called "unethical". The "pro" thinkers are not perturbed by this for they know that the basis of "con" arguments are a wrong conception of human "life" and an unfounded idea that such life is extra terrestrial. Yet, some people argue that to say that life does not begin even at the sixteenth or even the twentieth week is too hard to digest because "viability" alone cannot be the real point of "life" in time. If it is taken that humans are so called when they are born, any born person on life saving machine for existence cannot be a person as they are like those unborn children who depend only on their mothers for existence. Thus merely "unborn" does not bereft conceptus of "life" or being called a "person in the making". As such at any stage of the conceptus, abortion is bad. As I have said, an extreme view would reject abortion even if some malady has been detected, though it is difficult to find one such view because no one is "con" to mother's life. At best they reject abortion of normal conceptus at any stage. However, for the "pro" view it is difficult to accept that the finding for "normality" is ever possible without constant monitoring of the stages of the conceptus, particularly at the sixteenth week for amniocentesis and other investigations which are vehemently opposed by the "con" thinkers because they fear (sometimes truly) that life is terminated for "sexual determination". "Pro" thinkers believe that we cannot have unnecessary fears of unethicality such as aborting the girl child and thus stop tests for detecting grave life threatening defects because for all of us normal child and normal mother, both are important. This squabble is particularly important for the Indians as we cannot deny both that there is rampant female infanticide after conducting tests for sex determination and that there is undue death of carrying mothers and babies for several biological maladies.

One interesting question is raised by the "con" supporters, they ask: "If we are still groping for a pertinent scientific reply to what is "life" and when it begins after conception, is it not rational to accept that any state after confirmed conception is able to give birth to a human life, and, therefore, it is ethical to be respected and not killed?" This is very interesting as these amounts to some defeat for the theory of "soul" because we are equally groping about the entry of something like this for "life" to commence. More interesting is to notice that the scientists and the religious men are relentlessly pursuing for proving their thesis, and for that reason the call is for acceptance for "soul" thesis which is itself under scrutiny. How far does its acceptance for convenience work? Is it ethical to accept something just on the ground that something has not been proved as yet? What do we 'prove' any way? "Life" is just a conception, a biological one which stands clarification of meaning within the broad field of that subject. How does "soul" and "God" come in such inquiry? And the biological science has its own definition, which does not uniformly agree that life is any state after conception. Why should non-scientists argue about the validity of a scientific thesis on non-scientific grounds? Is it not blatant category-confusion?

The stiff scientific resistance to a non (or 'un') scientific explanation of "life" abolishes further "con" arguments for sanctity of value of life. If the problem of "life" is really undecided, it is not that we accept any state of conceptus as 'living' rather, it should be rationally accepted that any state of conceptus cannot be explained emotively. Hence, there is no point in projecting states of conceptus as "innocent" which for no fault should not be aborted by medical men, and that none of the rights and privileges enjoyed by mothers "override" those of the conceptus not to be aborted. In fact, using the concept of "rights" of conceptus is a further misconception because it is not a "living being". But there are problems say the "con" thinkers, because today the environmentalists realize that even rocks enjoy certain rights. A lump of cells may it be, an early conceptus does enjoy right to live unharmed in mother's body because it is not they (the rocks or tadpoles or zygotes) who cry for rights, but we do because any disrespect to even rocks amounts to environmental catastrophe or to tadpoles amounts to imbalance or to zygotes amounts to the "domination" of a killer instinct in men, most disrespectful to women and unborn fetuses. It is much like Nazi conception of mass genocide after legalization of abortion. Well, this is something bogus for the "pro" viewers for the charge extends from biology to sociology. Even if it is true that rocks and tadpoles are protected for their rights we have imagined, conceptus does not have one because there are no adverse effects on environment or on mothers or on humanity at large. Many societies (non-Nazi) have legalized abortion for social reasons like population boom, without any idea of mass genocide or disrespect to women and unborn. Sometimes affluence is bad, as population burst in India is to the Indians and here medically terminating early conceptus may be ethically good rather than bad for the masses. No one here till date legalizes girl child to be aborted for that reason because it has been always stated that medical termination of pregnancy is desirable in early stages when we are *under a veil of sexual ignorance*. Equally true is that at a later stage, even if a girl child is found to come to existence with some grave biological defects amounting to threat to mother's life, no one is so emotional to illegalize abortion. The problem is that the socio-political reasons for Nazis to legalize abortion are not the same for the non-Nazi governments. The objectives of legalizing abortion in a civil society does not presume emotional things such as encouragement of genocide but the objective of Nazis was exactly to kill someone nurturing in a Jewish womb. However, the "con" view retorts saying that factually, in India, for instance, the Nazi mentality to abort for either population control or for female birth control has grown in the recent times owing to legal termination. However, this is confusion because what is legalized is not for terminating girl child in any case but for population control.

The ethical questions about this matter unfold for us the possibility of a lively debate. We will most likely take up this debate at length but not before we had some more questions for us. The "con" viewers try to strike at the beehive by throwing another question to the medical men. They ask: What if abortion procedures you have invented are themselves against the health of the women who carries a conceptus? Is it not unethical to intrude into women's privacy by harming their organs for abortion even if someone has consented to such procedure? Should the doctor, who is supposed to know best about the biological well-being of humans go for some *medically dangerous procedure*? Let us suppose that the case of abortion is not urgent, that is, more of a non-life threatening one, why should doctors prefer it? Any method such as D&C, uterine aspiration, hysterectomy, saline abortion and self-induced abortion have their own health hazards, why should someone knowingly go for it even at an early stage? Are women mere objects for them? All is well said, but the "pro" thinkers argue that the medical researches are finding out better means to safer abortion in consented cases. The likely effects are normally explained to the parties, which override some dangers for greater benefits. In fact, not having such procedures may be more dangerous for mankind. Moreover, at later stage abortions, it may be more painful if not impossible. Hence, better take some risk than not. When something helps us more, it should be done or else why take medicines after reading its side-effects?

Another stone in the beehive is thrown by "con" people is this: Though there are dangers in a women conceiving and going through pregnancy to give birth to a child, modern medicine has tried to minimize suffering for successful delivery. Hence, rather than termination, medical science strives for safer birth. If, in this course, a child is unwanted or is found to be deformed, there are alternatives to abortion. For instance, there are people who want to adopt these babies and take great care of them. Even unwanted children are well nurtured by caring homes or governmental institutions. Hence, overlooking all viable alternatives there is no point in aborting fetus, it is unethical. The "pro" viewers retort that unwanted and deformed babies might live a miserable life for no fault of their own, they will ever lead life in great mental pain owing to social neglect and at times may be a matter of great social and governmental burden in the face of already booming population. Moreover, the "con" thinkers do not think seriously about the possibilities of grave genetic defects and even deadly diseases which they carry from parents when they are born which becomes another problem for the family and the society. Is it not ethically good to terminate them before they become palpable problem for the society at large? I have already said that not all "con" thinkers are obstinate enough to accept the truth that 'safe pregnancy' would mean the possibility of a healthy birth that is, at least not threatening to life of many people in society.

The point of "consensual sex" is extremely important when we listen to the "pro" and "con" questions and their replies. The point is that every normal male and female human should bear the legitimate responsibility to rear children as consequence of consensual sex. In such cases economic and social excuses does not matter much. To the problem posed by the "pro" people that post conception and after birth there are many financial and social burdens which many people fail to face and for that reason unwanted child may be aborted, the "con" people argue that if some people do not know the consequences of free consensual sex and if they are not ready to face them after birth, it is their fault, which is ethically unpardonable. Hence, no one can abort just because they are too poor to rear a child. Normally such people should not have too many children and if at all they have one, they should face it. In case of free consensual sex these people should be reminded of the use of contraceptives, which they overlooked. But this is a mistake on their part and any social fear after conception leading to abortion is morally unacceptable – foolish acts in themselves, unethical at times. The "pro" people have their own reasons in this regard as most of the time they rely on the emotional and accidental aspects of consensual sex. Poor people or anyone else often fails to suppress the natural sexual urges in the free consensual sex, when it is but natural to fall prey to accidental conception. In such cases, looking at the social, financial and other aspects for abortion is ethically justifiable, they say. This is much stronger in case of conception after rape because here the element of accidence overwhelms consensual act though sex is common in both cases. The "pro" people think that in such cases, social, economic and personal fears are natural and justified to great extent, which becomes the ethical ground of abortion. When some acts of sex are unwanted, their unwanted consequences are equally undesirable; hence, abortion is justifiable. The "con" argument questions whether or not in the accident the conceived life had any fault? If 'no' is the reply then it should continue in the process until birth and there are possibilities of law being able to nab the rapist to equitably punish him to rear the child or marry the girl or even arrange for a home to rear up.

One so-called strong argument by the "con" theorists is that opposition to abortion is not merely due to the fact that the conceptus is live but that the conceptus belongs to a live human. Hence, human conceptus enjoys a special status by being member of the human species, which enjoys a unique advantage in biotic community. Hence, it is unethical to destroy conceptus by deliberate means like abortion. However, the "pro" theorists do not like such "speciesism" and call for the unethical attitude to be eradicated from our mind. For them, being a human fetus we have no right to non-killing if needed as many other animals along with their conceptus are killed for many other reasons. Whether or not speciesism is itself ethical is one important question for the debate. However, the spirit of the "con" group is not dampened as they think that species has unique sentient features at the conceptus stage, for which it is unethical to kill because "sentience" is key to the enjoyment of moral status of the conceptus. What is crucial in being a sentient being is that humans feel pleasure and pain, which are respectively, inherently good and evil and as such respectively desirable and undesirable. Hence, any deliberate harm to the fetus causes irreparable pain which is ethically undesirable. Arguing further the "con" view holds that the human conceptus at the third trimester onwards does have such status of parts of functional brain such as responses to sensory stimuli that it arguably feels pain if aborted, and, therefore, unethical. Interestingly, for the "pro" people all this is testimony to avoidance of abortion at relatively later stages such as third trimester onwards but not at early stages. Hence, what they basically hold is morally good enough. Moreover, if "sentience" is the moral criterion for unethicality of abortion, not a single fly could be killed. Or, if flies would rapidly increase in numbers and thus some killed may be soon replaced, may not be justifiable in case of rapidly increasing Indians. Naturally, we have to look for any criterion other than sentience which enable humans more moral status than flies for not being killed. The "con" thinkers speak of "other criterion" which is "personhood", this amounts to several things, but what is relevant to the status of fetus and abortion is that qua persons we are just not agglomeration of bodily organs including brain and sense organs who have various feelings and sensations, we are rather persons having moral capacities to deliberate for good and right, choose and act. If this be so, much different from rabbits and even chimpanzees we need to consider the deliberate harm caused to an otherwise potent person in abortion. Hence, even if it is argued that early fetus or even a later one is not a "person", we are persons having moral concern for those likely to be a person like us if it is unabated. The "pro" people point out that even if it is true that we are morally conscious and fetuses are not, that conceptus likely to be born as near vegetables and morally non-responsive should be aborted on the basis of personhood. But there is a point, what do we do with vegetative persons infesting the world now? Do we kill them? Retorting back, one may say, well, the person is vegetative now after being so responsible moral agent, and, therefore, not to be killed. Moreover, living vegetables are incomparable to conceptus in many ways, in former case, we do not "abort", we "assist in ending life" (which is a glossed expression of "killing"). Certainly no medical man prefers "killing" as substitute for "aborting" because that ends them in a lock-up.

By this time I have said many things about the supporters of medical termination of pregnancy. We may put them together very briefly here as the view basing arguments on the biological conception of life as starting with birth, the biological need for ending unwanted, deformed and diseased children, the biological well-being of women, the social needs for moving out of trauma of rape and consensual sex leading to accidental pregnancy, the right to abort as part of responsibility to sexual act and most crucially the feminist view that women enjoy exclusive moral right to decide over pre and post-consensual sex consequences. As I have touched upon almost all "pro" arguments, it is important to briefly mention here the last one. The argument is that females like males enjoy equal rights over their body and sexual decisions. As such, they have every right over the conceptus after consensual or accidental sexual acts, and for that matter none of the associated males and females need to intervene in this matter.

Decision for abortion is one viable way to decide over the fate of the concept which is thus morally fine. Though another decision is not to abort, which will be equally fine on the part of the woman but she cannot and should not gloss its ethicality on clumsy non-biological grounds. This would amount to some kind of a paradox, which amounts to say that the only basis of either abortion or continuation of pregnancy is well-being of the woman concerned. Hence, "well-being" does not completely rule out non-abortion either. What it only asserts is that woman has right to abortion apart from the non-abortion though in any case other than the woman none is interested. But what does it mean to give equal sexual rights to men? In case of consensual sex, these poor people will not have any say in contraception perhaps, or, they do not have any say in selection for furthering procreation. What is so good in neglecting these people if "well-being" of woman is more often than not a matter of joint exercise in our society? What if a female doctor *suggests* conceived woman to not to abort for her well-being on biological grounds? So far we get it, she will do "whatever is best to her reason and conscience" but what is the surety of "best" and the validity of her "reasons" and "conscience", with all respect that she has a strong mind and heart to do so?

It is interesting to listen to feminists like Judith Jarvis Thompson to support the case of abortion on the basis of a particular conception of "right to life" which does not entail "a right to use the body of another person". This further entails that pregnancy owing to rape and incest call for abortion, which is ethical as well. No one should question (no male or female chauvinist), that the early 'conceptus being living or sacred or a boon (!) is unethical to abort because the woman who suffered a trauma in non-consensual hazardous sexual act should be ethical enough to bear a child. It is a matter of the woman concerned what to do with the conceptus because only she has the right over her body and her decision related to the sexual aspects of her body. Yet, it will be interesting to find out if a woman decides in favour of going through her pregnancy due to her profound religious nature. Is her decision regarding her sexual life still ethical on religious grounds? In one sense, it may be so, but in another sense, not so, but in any case her decision is the final one. But if we believe Thomson, the one ethical wisdom of the person is to abort it. This is total neglect to another option we have mentioned for a feminist. It is interesting to notice that the feminist argument holds good even in case of pregnancy owing to ignorance and failure of contraceptive measures. We may still ask Thomson whether or not neglect towards the consequences of post traumatic or accidental pregnancy is any good because equally true is that the best minds may not be pragmatic, injudicious, extra-emotional and even immature to decide the touted right and good for herself just as something has happened to her body and she has right over it. We all have right over our bodies but that does not mean that there is none in the world who would give me some ethical wisdom not to abort an unwanted fetus because certain 'consequences' of doing so would be bad and not good. Or, none would give ethical wisdom to abort the unwanted fetus for the bad 'consequences' it has. The theory of 'right' of Thomson in any case does not lead us to "necessary abortion" if the theory is not associated to a calculus of the consequences of "necessary abortion" in one case as different from other cases. Some queer questions might trouble Thomson further. Let us now come to the problem of ethic of abortion in relation to female feticide which is much graver issue in India. What would people like Thomson prefer in India when she finds that what she accidentally conceived is a "female"? One reply is that we do not have to wait for that time because for every feminist earliest abortion of conceptus is ethically judicious, though we have said that not every female is a feminist who prefers this option on some other grounds. The problem is that Thomson and we all should realize that human life, mind and emotions are all unpredictable though it is possible that one continues through a concealed pregnancy for some tough social reasons or owing to inaccessibility to abortion or due to its unaffordability to find that she has a girl child, but what after that? Or, what if she gets a boy child? Does she give some salt to the girl for infanticide as is a common practice to save her from further disrespect? Tougher questions are that if all facilities of abortion were there and still someone could not abort it early for several queer reasons of mind to find at some point that she carries a female fetus, does feminist prescribes abortion? Or, if feminism is not anti-male movement, does she prescribe abortion in case of a boy-child? In India, however, it is not feminists who face these problems, these are faced by umpteen women of towns, cities and villages. Abortion is a problem for common females of India who are challenged for tough decisions in the midst of a social cobweb knit by men and women around them who are in one word, "chauvinists". Here females are faced mostly by "female feticide" even if she carries through a pregnancy of other consensual or traumatic sex. Here females are faced for abortion at the risk of going to quacks or to obtain crude unscientific methods threatening to life. The problem is what is the ethical validity of our health care takers lending a support to female feticide medically? The problem is what is the ethical validity of our health care managers and policy-makers not lending support to poor women to either prevent such feticide or prevent abortion at any stage? To my mind, all churnings are good enough on paper—all talks of rights, consequences and sanctity of life would be of no value if we do not pose ethical challenges to our health care takers and health care policy-makers to come out of their comfort zone to face these questions.

QUESTIONNAIRE

1. What is the value of "human life" to you? At what stage of gestation do you think that "life" is induced and what relation do you see between the gestating women and the induced conceptus in her?
2. In the light of what you have said, try to evaluate the cases of medically aborting conceptus at the earliest state possible and at a much later state (when practically feasible) both with regard to consensual sex and forced sex.
3. How do you look at the moral aspect of tests for determination of sex of the fetus and those for any biological defects of the fetus? Now evaluate your position with regard to medical termination of pregnancy.
4. Do you think that a woman and her associates have moral right to be informed about everything (including sex) that has been revealed in tests conducted on fetus?
5. What is ethical in allowing early abortions of conceptus under a veil of sexual ignorance in India? Or, is it unethical to you?
6. What should be the legitimate moral rights, obligations and duties of the gestating women, physicians and other health caretakers with regard to the decision about continuing with pregnancy or terminating it?
7. Is it ethically just to transfer governmental duties and obligations of decisions and actions for abortion after required tests to private institution?
8. Is it ethically just to transfer governmental responsibilities in case of abortion to untrained people for women in villages and women of weaker sections?

9. Suggest some decision-making rules in this regard for our health care takers and policy-makers.

With this we come to the end of this discussion. As I have already said, I shall briefly take up the case of *ethic of euthanasia* in the Indian context when it comes to taking life medically because it is till date an insignificant ethical ripple in Indian Diaspora. Nothing is perhaps as ambiguous as the sense of "euthanasia" because it may refer to either allowing death or mercy death or assisted suicide or mercy killing. "Allowing death" amounts to some kind of lackadaisical medical intervention or complete *non-intervention* in care and cure of a sick person to let the person die a natural death at the request of the person or his associates or both, which is also corroborated by the health caretakers for it is pragmatic to not act heroically or do anything not worth doing. This is medically speaking, a not so uncommon feature. When, for instance, someone has been suggested to go home and wait until death by stopping frequent dialysis and allied measures to save life. This is not neglect or failure of the scientific Diaspora rather, one wise step to stop where continuing costly treatment is of no use. Euthanasia is not exactly this form of 'non-intervention' because in its case there is *positive intervention* to end life in a scientific and as much painless way as possible with or without the consent of the sick person but not of healthy ones. Medically speaking, allowing healthy persons to die is not possible if the person is not isolated for a systematic torture for continuous lack of food, water, pure air and medicines but all these tortuous ways are not within the science itself. If some trained people obtain it, they will be permitted by law for gross violation of medical principles and objectives. Interesting is to notice that if systematically death is "allowed" in health care institutions after admission or if there is deliberate slow-down in attending the sick person, it may be equally illegal and objectionable, for which there are some ways to punish as well. Heroic efforts to save life is not looked down, but slowing down is. However, these things may be nicely concealed in professional efficacy particularly if there are little or no checks by any agency, or if parties concerned agree to these measures within or outside the institution. The most fearful aspect is to allow death by sheer negligence without any agreement which is also punishable. In any case, we cannot say that illegal aspects of allowing death alone make it euthanasia because the key to distinction is "active medical engagement in taking one's life for a so-called good of the sick person killed". Mercy death is still farther from euthanasia for it is *not* taking life through active medical intervention for any good *perceived by the treating community* rather, a medical aid to do good as perceived by the sick person alone. Hence, what we now get in terms of "euthanasia" is one active medical way to take a sick person's life for reasons deemed to be necessary and sufficient for the good of the sufferer as perceived by the sufferer and/or the attendants and the physicians. In this sense, euthanasia is close to "mercy killing" but *not* "mercy death", which is truly a form of suicide in medical assistance. We need not embark much on the illegality of mercy death for assisted suicide is almost globally punishable particularly if the assistants are registered doctors and nurses functioning in private and public health care centers. We are however, interested today in the legal aspect of euthanasia because after the Netherlands making it legal, it is hard to say that globally it is illegal. Most interesting feature is that stiff debates are raged to justify and unjustify the ethicality of both "allowing death" and "euthanasia". Comparing this to mercy death, its justification and refutation for ethicality is not so raging though it is not difficult to find persons suffering from terrible diseases at one point to urge for assisted death because it is his life and he has all right to end it at will with least suffering lest he is unable to do so in assistance. Our ethical concern is not about such suicide or over allowing death. We want to scrutinize the ethical questions in euthanasia or mercy killing.

The need for euthanasia and its ethical justification among physicians and attendants despite its legal obsessions is mainly owing to the concept of "brain death", that is, a condition in which a surely 'injured person's heart, lungs and vital organs have been activated but not the brain, for it has been irreversibly destroyed, calling the person at that point "medically dead", perhaps "pragmatically dead" as well. The point is not whether or not we "allow" him or her to die rather, whether or not despite other functions going nicely, we should still go for some such medical means to kill the person after consent of attending parties including persons of family and legal and other representatives. Very unlike allowing death, this is a wholesome "team effort" as if to end the life of the brain dead person though without his consent. Euthanasia is not restricted to "brain death" cases as we shall shortly find out. It is now more interesting to see that any question of "ought" or "should" in this case is not what is "medically desirable, right and just" rather what is "morally desirable, right and just", that is, what is right and just on certain moral basis and not merely practical basis. Much ethical heat is generated in euthanasia debate about such "basis". However, a proper evaluation of all this is possible when we have further consented "types" of euthanasia because moral arguments are not similar in case of all types of euthanasia.

Ethicists these days classify euthanasia as *voluntary*, *non-voluntary* and *involuntary*. In the first case, there is systematic medical intervention to take the life of a suffering person, hopefully in a stage of no-return to normalcy but not as vegetative as the brain death, that is, perfectly conscious to deliberate about his conditions and for a possible continuity and death. However, 'taking life' is in accordance with the deliberation of the person concerned might transcend a present "now", that is, it is not necessary that the ailing person "now" has given the physician a permission to take life rather, may have done so in the past when he or she was able to do so but "now" fail for certain disabilities of body and mind. This point is crucial in understanding the honest covenant between the physician and the patient in a written or oral form, which may be honoured at a point of time as deemed to be most "suited" by the physician and none else. This enables us finally to realize that the patient understands the "good" in dying, the physician "agrees", for that "good" outweighs the "evil" of suffering and subsequent death. However, the decision for death is not at patient's wish but doctor's prudence for that good. All these clarify that voluntary euthanasia is not exactly "assisted suicide" for in this case, we get an idea of the death at a present "now" in collaboration with the person wishing to die and the one who provides it systematically. As such "voluntary euthanasia" cannot be legally evaluated at par with "assisted suicide", nor can it be morally evaluated as in case of assisted suicide. "Non-voluntary euthanasia" is again a case of administering medical doses of lethal drugs or systematic withdrawal of medical aids to a vegetative patient as we have seen in case of brain death when the person had perhaps never thought of such way of dying in medical assistance, or have never consented in the past or the present, or have never wished to anyone close to him that if he ever has a fateful vegetative future, he be killed in such way. However, it is hard to imagine that even helping such people to die, a physician has not taken his or her associates or relatives in confidence fit to serve a legal purpose. Euthanasia is "involuntary" in typical cases of medical assistance amounting to death in which the person did have a wish to die or to give consent but never did so clearly for the person may not have been asked to do so or because preferred to continue living for some more time. It is perhaps "taking life" in an assumption on the basis of certain verbal reports provided by the patient or his parties at some time that had things become unbearable and not pragmatic, he or she would prefer dying. This is often the case when a conscious but critical patient is brought for treatment, wished she died for such and such reasons but withheld consent to face the music a little farther but others felt it is too much and when she went in a coma, snapped life sustaining system. It is very important to notice that if we evaluate all three cases of euthanasia for their "meaning", they make sense whether we have legally permitted it or not because under the clout and cover in our civil societies, any of these forms might exist, some of us know and others do not know. Hence, it is more important for us to discuss in our societies whether or not such acts are ethically desirable because that paves the way to a legal reconsideration of these acts or more strongly safeguarding for a likely flout of law. In Netherlands, the story should be the same though they have legally permitted it because they need not now debate on which form or forms are best rather, whether or not they continue it for such and such ethical reasons. In India, for instance, though we have not legally allowed any form of euthanasia, we openly discuss about its ethical validity and its legal obsessions, which makes a fresh challenge for our decision-makers to accept or rubbish it. It is further important to notice that when it comes to the ground reality of providing euthanasia to someone, we may do it in two ways: *actively* and *passively*; that is, we may push a lethal injection to end life or we may gradually stop medicines and life sustaining mechanisms. Active and passive euthanasia are thus "methodological" concerns for medical men. It is also important to notice that euthanasia does not necessarily need a law in our societies, we really have them since a long time but mostly in the non-voluntary and involuntary forms in active or passive fashions. Truly speaking, it may not necessarily need a doctor or a nurse because it is not difficult to find such cases in our families though in any case, they are silenced for social obsessions, legal measures and moral concerns. The question is, if euthanasia is there "outside" health care institutions as conducted by "outsiders", is it truly "euthanasia", or simply assisted suicide or homicide? The definition of euthanasia cannot be blurred if it really has to be debated for ethical right and good because mere social participation, that is, participation of the persons outside medical fraternity but aided medically, may not be sufficient to call it "euthanasia". So the looming questions of morality and legality are about "participation of medical men" and/or "common people". To my mind, the moral permission and legalization need both participants to act in tandem or else we have none to participate if deemed to be immoral and illegal. For me the sense of euthanasia as a moral debate is about its desirability of practice by medical men at proper places for just reasons which also include fixing responsibilities to common men at their respective places for the same practice. I do not find any reason why euthanasia will be a practice at our homes as conducted by non-medical men for any good moral reasons. This point I shall stress because much ambiguity about "euthanasia" is due to fact that it is anyone's affair. If it really is, it is profound mistake because non-medical men do not have any scientific, legal and moral authority to extend such favour or disfavour to living men because they had just reasons which are also morally acceptable. It is a tragedy if we conceive of a situation in the Netherlands where Tom and Dick push injections to kill their wealthy uncle who used to be a rich man but turned vegetative after leaving a will for their worthy nephews to cash on it. Is it not frightening that the Netherlands did all this without a medical and legal supervision? If they did not, what it is to "legalize" and "moralize" killing is not known to me. There is no scope for making the sense of euthanasia ambiguous by equating it to "suicide" and "homicide" though in India, as we now stand, it is a form of "homicide" as per law but there is an urge to change a vision or to modify law because there are certain arguments justifying its pragmatic and moral value. Hence, much heat is now generated in our countries, where it is a "homicide" to find for medical fraternity and for medical reasons, whether it is permissible or not. Heat is also generated in our countries to find out the ethical grounds of allowing it for the medical men at least under legal supervision. So we cannot be so obstinate as to trash the debate because stubborn legal snubbing turns out to be foolish at times or they may come out in flying colours, consolidating its legal position. Thus the moral debate should be continued. Thus we cannot throttle it.

Before moving deeper into ethical arguments about euthanasia, we should have a quick look at the Indian scenario because I have said that though the debate is a small ripple in our nation, it has made some impact on some thinking people in and outside the legal and medical fraternities. Let us speak of Kolavennu Venkatesh who died of irreversible muscular dystrophy without fulfilling his wish to donate his vital organs to save life in Hyderabad's Global Hospital having a specialty organ transplantation wing. Venkatesh filed a case in the Andhra Pradesh High Court seeking euthanasia on December 8 of 2004. Further on December 13, his lawyer incorporated a request for live donation of heart. Hence, it was studied and understood by a committee that he was not brain dead and live donation was not allowed under Transplantation of Human Organ Act of 1995, which however, allows only cadaver organs for transfer. Subsequently, the court refused Venkatesh's plea for euthanasia and live donation, and on December 17, he passed away. Honourable Court viewed that law does not allow us to die at will in the ways of either euthanasia or live donation of heart, which amounts to a special way to 'voluntary euthanasia' through donation. Justice N.C. Rangrajan, Retired judge of Andhra Pradesh and Madras High Courts observed in a paper that Venkatesh was properly served with justice as his appeals, when respected, led to a 'slippery slope' form ethicality to unethicality so to say because live organ transplant is not distinguishable from homicide on the part of the participants of the collaborative act. He also argued that certainly we have "right to life" that includes "right to be brought to life", "the right to be born", "the right to have one's life maintained", "the right not to be killed", "the right to save one's life" but not "right to terminate one's life" and "the right to have one's life terminated". The "negative" aspects of "rights" regarding "life" enable courts to rule out requests for suicide, live organ donation and euthanasia. This also consciously and codifically bars doctors to do the same in the light of Hippocratic Oath. It is also *immoral* he says to prolong one life at the cost of another life. The can of ethical worms thus bursts for an offering to fall prey to it. But an Editorial in the same newspaper after quoting a famous verse from *Gitā*, which is a total misfit here, argued that Venkatesh had every right to shed off any of his parts because the whole was so "tattered". It argued that "without a right to death" the constitutional guarantee to "right to life" has no sense. In fact, the "right to life" includes or rather implies "right to die". Any intervention of the state in matters of death would be thus an immoral entry into private affairs. Moreover, the IPC has expanded its entry to suicide already (Section 309) but "euthanasia" is undecided for debate. So did the ruling come against an idea of "suicide" as Venkatesh's request could be learned by us? However, we learn that he requested for euthanasia and live donation of organs and nothing more. It must be that for "live donation" we had a law and thus enforced in this case but what about "euthanasia"? Was Venkatesh's counsel unwise to incorporate request for "transplant" rather than suggesting another way for mercy death? Did the request made everything ambiguous? Or, was it that "euthanasia" was taken as "request for assisted suicide", which, however, must be a misconception? So, a flow of queries, moral ones mostly, mixed with prickly pragmatics invite us more. Truly, the door was open for a debate as we did not have a clear code or a ruling about euthanasia. The debates harped on Venkatesh's ill fate for he did not get justice just because people are obsessed with "killing" as a crime, which "euthanasia" is not, and because the science stood stupid on the ashes of an early Greek called Hippocrates. Why should a medically vegetative, a useless life be not ended for another greater good or at least a potent possibility of it when even religion allows "killing" if intentions are pure? Why should law be an instrument of abuse when it is so unethical? What interests me most is that "people", non-philosophers, non-medical and non-legal ones, started speaking about the ethic of euthanasia. But the law appears to be steadfast because in April 1994, Justice B.L. Hansaria and R.M. Sahi in a Supreme Court judgment had already maintained that there is no point in equating "right to die" and "euthanasia" because in the case of "euthanasia", a third person aids in killing another person, for which he is not allowed by the law. With this background, let us move to a battery of questions emerging from the cases of *active* and *passive* euthanasia.

We have seen that voluntary, involuntary and non-voluntary euthanasia are either actively or passively done. The toughest question asked by the opponents of any form of euthanasia is, why should we at all debate for morality and legalization of some such practices like this one, which drags us to a slippery slope of genocide? Now, this question as I have just mentioned takes euthanasia as homicidal or at least leading to that state and finally to "genocide". The most popular way to compare this act is with Nazi act, a profoundly immoral act to allow thousands to die at the hands of a few out of sense doctors, nurses and freak people or criminals as Jews had in the hands of mindless Germans. Now, why on earth should every homicidal act lead to genocide? And why should euthanasia be Nazi-act, which is in reality, a "racist" act than a non-racist act as euthanasia? It would be such act if and only if a clout of doctors and nurses decide to 'take life' or 'let die' for only one race or else euthanasia is not Nazi-act. May be "Nazi-act" is only one metaphorical way to remind the supporters of euthanasia that if some of us are allowed to 'take life' or 'let die', we grow a "killer instinct", extremely anti-human or better said, anti-suffering human, which further slides us to the grave of genocidal instincts, that is, we would be extremely *intolerable* at the face of all sorts of human miseries, even those of our erstwhile dear ones for we have lost all respect for their lives. Is this not Nazi-act in this sense? The supporters might retort saying that such fertile imagination presupposes wrong things right because no able psychiatrist would find a thin chance from killing or letting one die for biological reasons in some cases to turn a killer first and then a mass killer. Well, there is point here. Are butchers killers? Is it true that any act of killing makes us "killers" by instinct? If this is not true, killing some people does not make us "killers". But opponents might still argue that all butchers are "killers" and euthanasia cannot be glossed by "letting die" or "taking life" as substitutes to "killing". Well, let us put aside "butchers" first because goats do not "allow" them for a *kārmic nirvāṇa* voluntarily, but what about non-voluntary and involuntary euthanasia? Who "allowed" people to be seen as goats in such cases? And who "allowed" people to see goats as vegetables?

The moral debate about non-voluntary euthanasia in active or passive ways is much stiff as we now assume. If a person did never choose to be killed, why should he be killed in a comatose state after an accident or be killed if he is conscious but not self-conscious? Why should a person's life depend on those who do not have right over his life? Moreover, why should some such things be done in our society which trigger fear among old, weak and debilitating people and even youthful, risk taking people that if they have not yet chosen to die, they will meet the fate by virtue of other's decision when time so comes? What is then so morally good to decide for other's death? Counter question will be, who can cure a diabolic sceptic? Why should we be so sceptical about our turning to be a vegetable or meet an accident and lull in coma? Even if biologically we deliberate of a day of coma, what is morally good to not accept that we should die peacefully than linger on the shoulders of others? Almost same patterns of questions might be asked when we come to involuntary euthanasia, though in this case the opponents might press on the point of immorality more on the ground of one's conscious states and well deliberated stand to continue living than dying which might have been his or her previous option. In any case then, the continued act to "bear pain at its worst" is a testimony to "urge to live" than "urge to die", which is an indirect way to suggest even in a comatose state what the person finally would have preferred – clearly, not to die at other's hand but in nature's course. Added to this is our beloved "God" whose sons and daughters we are, and who redeems us from our "urge to die" when in pain. As the life is His gift, why should we be so ungrateful and immoral to allow a petty man to take it? The world, however, is very funny for the supporters of involuntary euthanasia because empirical proofs lead them to umpteen cases when one who urged to live in pain decided to die when in pain in real life, and that directly suggests death, whether in coma or not in coma. Equally funny is "God" for these people whose children we are. Well, our biological parents are our gods who gifted us "life" even if there is some debate about "God". But what is moral in thinking that the "gift" was so noble as if we had no right to decide over its fate? Does the donor have natural right to handle the gift when it is too tattered to be handled any further? As regards to other's, "taking" it is not a problem because the gift had no biological value to be saved at *any cost*. What these supporters amount to say, may be now extended to "voluntary euthanasia" as well because it boils down to our *freedom*, *autonomy* and rights to decide on the way we should die. One addition to this is, some responsible people also enjoy some moral right to decide the way we should die when it is most needed. In this case then, the notion of "rights" takes a peculiar extension as does the notions of "costs and benefits". Any way, the field of moral debate is ripe for us to enter into it. Take this questionnaire if you wish.

QUESTIONNAIRE

1. Why is human life valuable to you? Whatever value it may have, it is mortal, and at some physical states we wish, we died and someone helped us in doing so. What is immoral in such wish or fulfilment of such wish by others?
2. Is it sensible then to speak about "right to die", "right to allow others to die" and "right of others to let us die"?
3. Do physicians and nurses have certain obligations? What are they? Do they have some duties? What are they? Is it obligatory and duty on their part to take life or let one die?
4. Why could there be a moral debate about voluntary, non-voluntary and involuntary euthanasia when law does not allow euthanasia or does allow euthanasia? Is it at all a moral issue?

5. Do you think that India has just laws in dealing with euthanasia of any form in and outside hospitals? If you answer is in the negative, suggest changes, and if in the positive, assert whether there should be further changes.

With this we come to the end of considering value-laden practical problems about life and death but here I may be excused to not to discuss what I have myself found in discussions arranged by me, though pro and con arguments and the questionnaire at the end of each sections gives ample idea about what go on in such debates. The most interesting thing is about "consensus", and I shall leave readers wondering perhaps by disclosing at least the truth that our wise people could not trash IVF, Cloning, Abortion, Euthanasia and Killing Animals in course of Researches, but having said so, I must be honest to mention that they could not trash some very strong points of not doing such things as well. Thus, what follows is "consensus" about doing all these in extremely cautions ways or better said, in restricted ways. It also opens a can of further moral debate for us for there is no complete satisfaction in intersubjective corroboration debates. Yet all this exercise is sensible if we really mean to jump in such interesting debates and not leave them aside. For our health care professionals – "Come out of your comfort zone".

NOTES

1. Robertson, John A., "IVF, Infertility and the Status of Embryos" in T.L. Beauchamp and Le Roy Walters (eds.), *Contemporary Issues In Bioethics*, Wadsworth, Belmont, p. 636.
2. *Ibid*, p. 645.
3. Sherwin, Susan, "Feminist Ethics In Vitro Fertilization" in T.L. Beauchamp and Le Roy Walters (eds.), *Ibid*, pp. 646-47.
4. Ibid, p. 649.
5. *Ibid*, p. 651.
6. *Ibid*, p. 652.
7. Winston, Robert, "The Promise of Cloning for Human Medicine", *British Medical Journal*, 314, 1997, p. 914.
8. Gutman, Huck, "Biological Confidence Game", *The Statesman*, Kolkata edition, 10.09.2001, p. 7.
9. Vlasak, Dr. Jerry, reported in *The Statesman*, Kolkata edition, April 1998, p. 24.
10. Singer, Peter, *Practical Ethics*, Cambridge University Press, Cambridge, London, 1993, p. 93.

11. *Ibid*, p. 99.
12. *Ibid*, p. 104.
13. Regan, Tom in T.L. Beauchamp and Le Roy Walters (eds.), *op cit.*, p. 493.
14. *Ibid*, p. 493.
15. *Ibid.*
16. Cohen, Carl in T.L. Beauchamp and Le Roy Walters (eds.), *Ibid*, "Do Animals Have Rights?", *Ibid*, pp. 495-501.
17. *Ibid*, p. 495.
18. *Ibid*, p. 498.
19. Callahan, Daniel, *Abortion, Law, Choice and Morality*, McMillan, New York, 1970, p. 44.

6

Conclusion

We have seen so far what biomedical ethics consists in but we have to find out now whether this entire craze in our times is merely short-lived or has a bright future. Talking about the bright future or prospect of bioethics, it depends on the amicable coexistence of biology, medicine, law and ethics; the proper methodology of teaching ethics and bioethics; and the participation of public in the resolution of bioethical issues, which becomes crucial in teaching bioethics as well. I believe that we have got some idea about all these three things in the earlier chapters because time and again we found that biomedicine is full of some such problems which are not specific to that field alone because these practical problems raise stiff questions of ethical and legal importance, which we cannot avoid without being both callous and unethical. We have also seen that the common men have something to say about a number of biomedical problems because these problems being closely associated to ethicality and legality, take moral beings into serious consideration. This amounts to say that certain biomedical issues ask for the participation of the public, not only those who are scientifically trained rather those fraught with many problems emerging out of biological and medical decision-making and actions. Such decision-making and subsequent actions of the bio-scientists often stir the minds of the legal experts, policy-makers and law-makers in our society, who are parts and parcels of the "general public" because we cannot deny that they too are affected by several biomedical decision-making and actions. On the other hand, the bio-scientists do not live an isolated life and they hardly assume that they should remain absolutely cut-off from general public decisions and actions as well as legal and governmental decisions and actions. In fact, many individuals, groups, and social, legal, legislative and executive decisions and actions influence biomedical decisions and actions to a great extent. Hence, we thought it practically and ethically just to accommodate the public in the course of the resolution of a number of practical biomedical issues ethical and legal questions in a model called "intersubjective corroboration". The transversal nature of biology, medicine, ethics, legality and public policies press us to accommodate this model of ethical resolution of the bioethical problems. Perhaps we have not thus far commented on the role and the value of corroboration of views, a model down to earth with regard to *teaching* ethics and biomedical ethics. Perhaps we were not explicit about the role and value of 'teaching' ethics and biomedical ethics in the glorious prospect of both ethics and biomedical ethics. We have to take these tasks in some more details, but not before we find something more interesting about the close relationship among biomedicine, ethics and law.

Biomedical scientists as we now understand are not alien people living in closed chambers, cut-off from public life. They are no demigods or people acting as gods, having no interest in what is going on in the society and the world around them. They are very much the common public having some specific training for the *general biological welfare* of other people like them, who are equally important as they themselves are. Any biomedical decision and action cannot transcend public life, and for that matter, public affairs and public policies. Truly speaking, such decisions and actions cannot transcend the currents of politics, economics, religious faiths, common morality, prejudices, obsessions, ethics and legality. Biomedicine is thus greatly motivated by common sense morality and ethics on the one hand and legality on the other hand. We must say that morality, ethics and legality are important factors motivating institutional and public policies because such policies are vital to public life or public affairs which are mainly governed by the conception of the "good over evil produced in such life or such affairs". Both ethicality and legality (to a great extent) are thus concerned about the production of the good of the public and as such keep close watch on some specific decisions and actions which either contributes to or disparages the production of such good. In this sense then, the institutional and public policies regarding public health care, crucial to the good of public life, should be under the ethical and the legal scanner. Hence, we have to accept the truth that biomedical decisions and actions, which are closely related to public well-being are motivated by as well as kept in such control by institutional and public policies and as such by ethicality and legality. Clearly, therefore, a "policy decision" and subsequent action by the public health caretakers cannot transcend the legal and moral scrutiny but we have to be careful about the use of "morality" here because there is a lot of ambiguity in the free use of "ethicality" and "morality" by virtue of our literary freedom to do so. What is in reality meant that "policy decisions" are motivated by our common *ethical concerns* of the good, just, right and desirable not by our traditional or dogmatic *moral opinions*. Let me discuss about this point which I think is very crucial in an understanding of biomedicine's closeness with ethics and law rather than morality, customs and traditional rules and codes. The readers of *The Primer* (vol. 1) do have an idea of such things, but for a better understanding here, we may produce it here differently. What I was stressing in the entire work is *not* that the public moral opinion, which amounts to the customary, traditional and orthodox opinions about good, right, just, desirable, duty, obligation which are important in the resolution of the value-laden practical problems, rather I was stressing on the *ethical probing* of the public (including the scientists) regarding the value-laden practical problems. It is important to understand that what I call, "ethical probing" is much different from "moral probing" because "ethical probing" apart from other things is systematic probing on many moral beliefs, faiths, opinions, traditions and customs as well. Ethical probing, truly speaking is also a systematic probing on one or more moral beliefs and opinions. Hence, ethical probing is in one way a critique of morality and of itself so that we come more and more closer to an understanding of the *bases of evaluation* of what is good, just, right, duty and obligation for the health care experts, the legal experts, the law-makers, the executive and the common people whose biological welfare we are trying to attain. In this sense then we do not stick to several moral customs, which have become fixed or orthodox and thus obsessions in our societies, and for that reason we choose to shed off such moral faiths and beliefs regarding health care issues. For instance, we have *moral obsession* to not to donate our vital organs after death for different *non-moral reasons*, mostly so-called religious ones or metaphysical in nature, but *we* constantly probe *ethically* on such "morality" prevalent in us even today so that greater biological good is possible. Here, the stress on "we" is due to the fact that "ethical probings" are not restricted to a class, the class of ethicists so to say because such things are not restricted to "knowledge of academic ethics" consisting of normative theories like teleology, deontology and so on. It is also not restricted to a course in ethical justification either, rather the constant participation in public affairs and in the resolution of value questions troubling the public life. This is possible, as I have said owing to our being members of ecological community and remaining sane headed therein. Our picking of moral customs, codes and habits in society is just as natural as picking up a religious affiliation but gradually we grow a habit to probe such habits, even our religious affiliations; similarly, we become ethically conscious about the should or the ought of decisions and actions without being officially either a deontologist or a teleologist, we thus gradually probe on our moral affiliations and ethical affiliations. We find ourselves perfectly at home in uttering wise words of welfarism, benevolence, beneficence and so on when we are faced with value-laden biomedical issues. We need not conceal the truth that even though many of us ably transcend prevalent or customary morality, soon fall in its trap, or that many of us transcend it and stick to ethical views which they find to be more reasonable to hold. To our great astonishment though, non-academic views on ethics or ethical probing are as good as any deontologists or teleologists or any official ethics we learn so far because all these never dropped from the blue in a wise man's mind. The wise men have uncanny ethical acumen than we have to systematize and shape such ethical conceptions to a "theory" and its "justifications". Interesting is to notice that *our* uncanny ability to *talk ethically* beyond being merely "moral" is revealed only in *association* with the public and not alone because people's ethics is not "academic", it is in itself not a theoretically based effort, it is predominantly practical or dynamic within public life and public affairs. Hence, we may now conclude that we are concerned with biomedical ethics and not biomedical morality. Biomedical ethics is not necessarily and sufficiently principlistic or theoretic. Biomedical ethics is thus sensible in the broader context of public life and public affairs, it is not sensible merely as a moral scrutiny of biological affairs and theoretical ethical scrutiny of biological affairs.

Now this "ethical scrutiny" of biomedical affairs is broadly speaking a part of production of good over evil through good policy formation as well as reviewing good policies formed. Bioethics, therefore, takes serious interest in the ethical *evaluation* of those policies, which are sets of normative, enforceable guidelines governing our biological decisions and actions *accepted* by the private and the public bodies, institutions and organizations; for instance, the hospitals, the judiciary, the legislative and the executive for a greater good. Biomedicine is thus closely related to ethics and laws pertaining to the *biological justice* in the human society in the primary sense and in the non-human society in an extended sense. There is no doubt however that formation of policies in public affairs such as biomedical affairs is an extremely complex matter, which is, as I have said, closely related to culture, religion, politics and economics. Hence, we should be careful about over simplism in this regard because ethical resolution of biomedical impasse cannot be itself sufficient if it disregards the socio-economic and political undercurrents that influences the problems and their resolution to a great degree. We need not forget that encouraging multinational companies in India in the field of health care does not only face ethical crises; such encouragement has close connection with the crisis in political and economic decisions regarding health care. Equally true is that any such political and economic decision calls for careful ethical scrutiny for its desirability. In the real-world situation therefore, ethical discussion cannot be devoid of cultural, political, economic and legal discussions, but the "ethic of multinationals' participation in health care" is always unique "ethical probing" or "ethical talk" about public health care decisions in a nation or a state, which decisions are social, political and economic decisions under the banner of a body of well-framed and accepted legal rules. It is due to this that we always take care of the ethical-legal constraints of any decision about public health care taken by either governmental or private bodies.

All this brings ethics and law together in the rescue of biomedical trifles. It is well said that biomedicine saved ethics from being dull theoretic enterprise but we also find that ethics and law in reality has saved biomedicine from many troubles. It is, therefore, in bad taste to prove that medical termination of pregnancy is "doctor's affair, let them be undisturbed", because doctors are social people, they are the people whose decisions affect us greatly either positively or negatively and they cannot be left alone to do whatever they like with the suffering lot. The very idea of "leaving them undisturbed" is unethical and illegal for "leaving" has a distinct sense of "chauvinism" or "being sacrosanct". Every medical man has to abide by certain laws and ethical decisions if they are truly social people, though there is no doubt that these responsible people can always debate whether or not certain laws need correction and whether or not certain ethical decisions about biological welfare were at all ethical. These people also enjoy the right to scrutinize whether or not some moral rules and codes need correction and whether or not some prevalent professional codes and rules carried on from generations have any value. Biomedicine is thus not a dull field of objective science; it has interesting things to do in connection with normative disciplines like ethics and law. If we come to know this, we find that the so-called fashionable medical code or codes for bio-scientists are not outcome of the churnings in bio-science itself rather are consequences of ethical-legal problems about several decisions, actions and policies inherent to the science. These codes are thus not "made by scientists" though they may be largely for them. Interesting is to notice that many such laws, codes and rules are not merely "for scientists" rather for the law-making and law-enforcing authorities as well. Hence, there is nothing such as "leaving bio-scientists alone"; they are obliged to the public, for their good under the guardianship of law and stand for ethical probing about their decisions, acts and the biomedical law itself. To quote Tom L. Beauchamp here will be good enough: "Law is the public's agent for translating morality into explicit social guidelines and practices and for determining punishments for offences. Both cases of law (judge made law expressed in Court decisions) and statutory law (federal and statutory and their accompanying administrative regulations) set standards for science, medicine and health care and these sources have deeply influenced bioethics"[1].

It is extremely important to eradicate confusion in our mind, which is fairly simple to do because we have said something about the relation of ethics, law and biomedicine. It is confusing legal evaluation of biomedical matters with moral evaluation of the same. In case of court law regarding medical disputes there is hardly any necessity of moral evaluation or moral probing because in such cases legal requirements are overriding so that "legal justice" could be done in the face of litigation among parties. Here we do not need moral theories or prescriptions even if such medically disputed issues are "value-laden" or raise distinct questions of ethical rightness and wrongness. In fact, certain "value-laden" issues do not stand in the way of either being independent of legal probing for some *ruling* or, independent of ethical probing for some *decision-making rules* for the professionals. It is interesting to notice, however, that the ethically probed and concluded matters might come in *conflict* with prevalent juridical law as established by the law-makers or confirmed by the court by virtue of evidences and instances. In this sense we cannot rule out an ethic of law itself, it is also not difficult to imagine a legal probing of ethically corroborated points because such things cannot safeguard itself as *absolutely good* in the eyes of law. The ethical challenge to law is often retorted by a legal challenge to ethical evaluation because the latter is based on different theses, whereas the former is based on other theses. Yet, we expect in this "conflict" that law need not disregard ethics and ethics should not disregard law because both are serious about value aspects in public life and public affairs. However, the problem that perennially remains are whether or not legally acceptable is also ethically acceptable and vice-versa. Take the case of Venkatesh for instance, he and we all knew that his death is a matter of little time to happen, though he wanted that he did not die without any contribution to society. So he desired for live donation of organs which also meant, he died instantly, which was thus regarded as a request for euthanasia. Now the law intervened because Venkatesh was "law-abiding", otherwise he would have simply asked someone to help him in donation, which he did not. He was seeking permission for other reasons as well, may be he knew that only law could revise itself by another legal ruling. Perhaps he did not want to go home and die because only hospital could fulfil his desire for death in donation and it is matter of law than anything else that hospital people just could not release him in that state though none of his desires could be fulfilled. Hence, there was a gruel battle among the sick, the physicians, the medical association and the law of the land. Now the hearing judge who had to 'rule' on this matter had no business to listen to complex ethical debates – the teleology, the deontology, the religious ethic and so on about euthanasia. What he was attending to is a battery of arguments, evidences and instances of practical nature which could justify why the present law about live donation amounting to the death of a nearly vegetative person was or wasn't desirable or in this sense, "just". So his effort was one of looking at established laws' veracity and nothing more. However, the ethical people have other ideas; they either think that what was legally ruled could be challenged for being *ethically right and just* or that everything remains unchallenged being ethically right and just. Ethically right and just depends on one or more *non-legal* standards such as teleology and deontology. But we desire that the legal and the moral should not be at loggerheads, rather accommodative. One instance of this accommodation is that though in India many of us shall harp on the ethicality of justice done to Venkatesh, we shall be equally careful to notice that many such requests should be under legal scanner for a lot of unethical practices in the name of euthanasia might spoil the ethic of the same practice. Is it not possible even in the Netherlands that the reversal of the law allowing euthanasia, under ethical pressures of peer groups, happens any day? It is possible because what has been corroborated now in the Netherlands as ethically just needed a legal back-up to be valid, which it did have but there are chances that ethical debates and legal problems change the course some time. Similarly, the barbaric laws of the Taliban era or those of the kings of India or even some of those in modern India were revised not for being unpragmatic rather being immoral and the peer groups strengthened the reversal of law for a long time now on ethical grounds. Rightly, therefore, Beauchamp writes that "The law appeals to moral duties and rights, places sanction on violators, and in general strengthens the social importance of moral beliefs. Morality and law share concerns over matters of basic social importance and often acknowledge the same principles, obligations and criteria of evidence. Nevertheless, the law rightly backs away from attempting to legislate against everything that is morally wrong."[2] Clearly, the prospect of biological ethics depends on the justification of it as something sensible to do within ethics having enough support from public life and legal opinions. Biomedical ethics being essentially dynamic in nature and not purely theoretic cannot be aloof about public's ethical and legal probes. This is important in further understanding of the value of participation of people and legal education in the curriculum of biomedical ethics.

But for that we have to first assert that biomedical ethics' bright future depends largely on *teaching* ethics and bioethics, which in turn needs participation of the non-medical people apart from the participation of experts in the fields of bioscience, law and ethics. Let us first consider the case of "teaching ethics and bioethics" to the core group, that is, the medical and the nursing students. Teaching "ethics" and "bioethics" are different things because the former consists of teaching wholesome ethics or a part of it for specific purposes to our medical and nursing students (henceforth, "core group"). In case of need of teaching wholesome ethics, we have to cover more and more relevant and important aspects in metaethics, normative, descriptive and virtue ethics, apart from a course in human values. In case of the need of teaching ethics partly, we should take up at least normative ethics, metaethics and courses in human virtues and values. Whereas in case of the need of teaching bioethics to our "core group" we have perhaps little choice to leave out one section or the other whimsically. However, for teaching the prospective nurses, a bioethics course need not cover everything that is prescribed for the prospective doctors. It is interesting to notice here that teaching bioethics or even ethics to our "core group" is one thing and to teach the same to "peer group" is another thing because in the latter case, our target group is nurses and physicians in active professional life not the prospective ones, for whom we have earlier used the word "students". In case of teaching ethics and bioethics to "peer group", it is not necessary to cover whatever is there in bioethics because the "peer group" may not be as organized and as free as the "students", that is, this group is relatively scattered, they need to be brought to an institutional set-up, to which they do not belong naturally or as a matter of right they do not claim such and such things ought to be taught to them. The core group is difficult to imagine without an institutional support; they are directly linked to a *future form of life* which is well-shaped in the institution in a systematic way keeping all practical needs in mind. Equally true is that the peer group does not come together without an institution taking some interest but here they are directly linked to shaping their *professional form of life* which was otherwise lacking or needed some refresher-booster. The difference enables the teachers to frame courses of ethics and bioethics best suited to both these groups. It will be overriding that "wholesome" courses of ethics and bioethics are offered first to the core group whereas some refresher courses for the peer group may be extremely restricted to suit present purpose. But this accepts the value of teaching ethics and bioethics in any case to our core and peer groups. Now here comes the difficult question: why should we attempt such things? This is to ask: who on earth gave teachers the sacred task to teach ethics and bioethics to the core and the peer groups, and for what reasons? No one has a doubt that any teaching programme should be well-thought out for the *objectives* first and then the curriculum that should follow. Hence, "objectives" of teaching clarifies the "reasons" for teaching ethics and bioethics to both the groups we are talking about.

It is important to remember here what I have already said (in *The Primer*) about *assumed objective* or objectives wrongly imagined by some of us and a *proper objective*, which is itself *ethical*. Let me briefly state what these things amount to in this context. In case of core or peer group we have to keep in mind that none in the world has the moral authority to assume that by teaching such and such things such and such people shall become "ethical" (as if they were unethical and we were sure of it and felt sorry for these poor people). Hence, none has the moral authority to imagine that they are benevolent teachers who would teach ethics and bioethics to ethicsless prospective professional nurses and physicians so that they become "ethical". It is a great misconception which the sophists had or any moral chauvinist has that the objective of teaching ethics and bioethics is to build great characters, and, therefore, great social work has been done. In fact, any amount of "classroom ethics teaching" to any group does not help in any way if one thing is not done, which takes us to the "proper objective" of ethics and bioethics teaching. We should aim at building a unique *cohesion* among students, professionals and teachers so that *theoretical* courses of ethics and bioethics are transcended for their potent practicability to enter into the realm of *practice* or application. We should be careful here to notice that after going through theories of ethics and bioethics, the learners are not prescribed for their "practice", that is, here the suggestion is not to use theories as means to resolve certain problems. Rather, our institutions should allow our learners to attend elaborate *moral discourses* to find out which theory or theories of ethics or bioethics, about which they are "theoretically aware" through courses emerges in our practical discourses. Hence, it is not teaching theory first and then applying it or not teaching theory aided by case studies first and then applying what we know rather *teaching theory parallel with our combined effort to have moral discourses* about bioethical matters. The entire process of learning needs common people to come nearer to us, people who may have different professional and occupations but are concerned with resolution of bioethical crises. This way what we theoretically know is *strengthened, extended* and *transcended*. It is "strengthened" because the practical venture leads to certain conclusions which go along with what theories propagated. It is "extended" because core, peer and teaching groups do not apply any one theoretical findings or some findings rather transverse moral opinions to come to a consensus, and because this group is constituted of many *non-scientists* and *non-ethicists* who have their moral opinions expressed about trifling matters and resolved them. It is "transcended" because pure theories are mixed with practical findings in the entire effort so that our critical acumen grows to evaluate them. We have to remember that this is true of teaching ethics and bioethics to our core and peer groups, which need not be in any case confused with teaching ethics to any other core or peer groups, for instance, to the students of teacher's training colleges or to the teachers of training colleges. The reason being that bioethics is a misnomer without "ethics" coming into it, and we have to first know "ethics" before we know "bioethics". Bioethics is an *ethical study* of some biological and medical issues, and not a biological and medical study of ethics for that is nonsense. Hence, in studying "ethics" we need to be careful that our core and peer groups are not only showered with the graces of great normative theories like Kantian deontology and Mill's utilitarianism and the like, rather they should grow power to *know* and *examine* them on a theoretical basis (as in metaethics) and on a practical basis (as in practical and professional ethics). Any attempt at the examination of ethical thesis in turn takes us to an effort for "cohesion" in moral discourses, which I have elaborated as *intersubjective corroboration*. Bioethics and its teaching are thus possible in the light of teaching ethics as well as bioethics having unique features apart from academic ethics if and only if "something is done" along with "something that is read". Bioethical teaching (as in ethics teaching) is essentially related to "practical jobs" in social contexts. It is somewhat like swinging like a pendulum from theory to practice and back to theory.

Now as I have offered an anti-climax regarding teaching ethics and bioethics for I have spoken what I feel but, I have further responsibility to find out and evaluate what many others hold in this matter so that I can justify or revise my position. Tony Hope of University of Oxford in his Editorial in *Journal of Medical Ethics* (24: 1, 1998) says that in the UK serious doctors have faced stiff challenges in medical institutions for setting up core curriculum in ethics for the doctors in particular because for some opponents the effort of ethics lovers is trivial or redundant or impossible. It is "trivial" because ethical impasse in medicine are rare, and when they come to the doctors, they find it trivial to learn ethics, it is so natural *for them* to resolve these impasse. For some, it is "redundant" for teaching ethics that has hardly any importance for a doctor treating an individual patient. Whereas for some, it is "impossible" because ethics is about our attitudes and character but not right or wrong theories and applications. Moreover, Mr. Hope mentions the charge of *moving in a circle* about this matter as teaching ethics begs effectiveness of a programme of teaching, whereas the said effectiveness begs teaching ethics. Yet, in the face of such scepticism, the General Medical Council of UK prescribes in depth special modules for medical students which consist of ethics and law. Thus core curriculum for *Tomorrow's Doctors* have been framed by virtue of a *consensus*, which Tony Hope thinks, answers the sceptical questions appropriately. The statement asserts of a core curriculum of ethics which is not merely "intellectually fascinating" such as ethic of cloning or surrogate mother or euthanasia (this I have also said at a place), rather those ethical issues should be discussed and resolved which are "clinically relevant" and "frequently in the practice of everyday medicine" so that we create "good doctors". Hence, "rights of children in health care" and "confidentiality" have more value for the curriculum and not for those mentioned above. Most importantly, this successfully answers the charge of "triviality", but not fully-as I believe because to this should be added that no one has urged our doctors (even prospective ones) to learn academic ethics and apply theories therein which do not "naturally" come to them. And what "they" (the doctors) think is so "natural" for them to resolve is fraught with problems because they act moral chauvinists who say: "I know my business, mind yours". But let me say that "My dear doctor, right to health care is a delicate issue, its ethical problem is not so naturally resolved by you or some of you for that needs many views to come together and corroborate", I would like to add further, the core curriculum suggested by the said Council stresses on "enabling students to think critically about ethical issues in medicine and to argue and counter-argue in order to contribute to informed discussion and debate". Mr. Hope truly says that he himself (and perhaps many others) encourage teaching ethics to prospective doctors involving *dialogues*. This enables us to move away from 'redundancy' of teaching ethics because such teaching does not even aim at tackling value crises of individual patients or those of doctors in case of a patient. When we are involved in arguments and counter-arguments regarding the resolution of value-laden problems, hopefully these problems are faced by the doctors, nurses and even the patient and his sympathizers who do not find resolution of one case but of many cases of similar nature. Most interesting is that the process is not everlasting because at the end of debate we find a way out of the impasse through a consensus. Hence, teaching ethics to our prospective doctors should rely not only on theoretical ethics rather involving in practical resolution of value crises in the field of medicine by considering one or more cases we find in our health care centers while we are at work. Apart from other advantages, in such cases, patients (some time) and his sympathizers might participate in or at least contribute indirectly in someway to the debate. The involvement of the public is great in resolving value questions and this in turn is good for teachers to demonstrate the way in real life our doctors are often placed and then it is better to remember the *consensus* views about the desirable features of the nitty-gritty of the practical aspects of treatment. This is not to imagine that for treating a case, every time a doctor has to ask for a debate and then decide, rather he should be aware of the ethical aspects involved in such cases for he has been through a *training in his life* which involved his moral views as well, and he is well-placed to know *what emerged in a consensus*. Here, I must add that such a teaching programme should be so flexible as to continuously and more and more widely appreciate value resolutions of ethical crises because there may be crystallization of disagreements over a period in some parts of our institutions or centers. Hence, the teaching methods we are conceiving is not static, there is nothing final in it for we are always moving with the flux of ethical arguments and counter-arguments – we do change when substantial consensus replaces a part of or whole of the earlier consensus. In any case, teaching ethics to our doctors should never fail to mention this counter-consensus before any other consensus has been reached. Enriching critical acumen of the participating prospective and trained doctors regarding ethical issues is possible only in this way, and this is a good way to make ethics interesting to the non-ethicists. From this we also get an idea that the charge of "impossibility" is unfounded as well because (as also Mr. Hope says), no one is interested among us to impose one or more normative ethical theory or theories on our students of ethics so that noble characters are made or some ethical issues are resolved. Ethics cannot be taught in this way because even our beginners quickly resists our persuasions or suggestions in such an artificial way because without being co-opted to any normative thesis, they are well-placed in value resolutions first and then come to know about the normative character of their own positions when teachers analyze further what their views amounts to in the context of academic ethics. To know ethics through an application transcends mere theory teaching. This is extremely good for those "non-philosophers" who are interested in ethics and bioethics in their career because they must know how important it is to know that non-co-opted people are themselves repositories of ethical knowledge. I must add that this way of teaching ethics at the beginning of a doctor's career or when they are refreshed in work-life enable them to see that when they themselves face value questions in practical life, they do not act as chauvinists, as ethical engineers, rather as good learners from the people around them, and from the many consensus reached through debates involving the public. Finally, about the charge of "circularity" it may be said that though the success of teaching ethics and medical ethics depends on the effectiveness of a core curriculum, the curriculum itself is not absolute or fixed, we have liberty to decide what suits best in our institutions or centers given the situations in which our prospective doctors, nurses or those coming for a refresher course is placed. In fact, the success of a core curriculum does not merely depend on teaching any course of ethics or bioethics, rather it depends on teachings based on a method stressing value of theory and practical involvement, which goes on revising, removing and incorporating things to be taught that gives any curriculum a "core" that is itself flexible and not absolute.

Whatever may be the details of the "core curriculum" formulated in the UK, we need not necessarily follow and adopt them in totality because I have just said that following something without any idea of need of our institutions is not a good idea. What is worth noting is that the "consensus report" finds a good role for teaching in a way of involvement when it comes to ethics and bioethics. In this context it is further important to ethically evaluate the practice of the use of patients in health care education. However, we must not have any confusion regarding *involvement* of patients in ethics and bioethics in health care education whenever that is possible and wise to do and *use* of patients in health care education. But what is so objectionable in "use" of patients when it comes to such noble and valuable things as health care education? Nobody really denies the practical value of the use of patients in health care education but the same may be objected to on "ethical grounds" when in the contemporary times the need of patients in such education is more intense owing to bridging the gap between theory and practice when we are particularly faced with theories which appear to be more imaginary than real. Hence, "involvement" of the public, including the suffering ones becomes all the more important when it comes to the *ethic* of teaching medicine by *using* sufferers. It is interesting to notice that such "involvement" has a distinct advantage, a moral one so to say, over an immoral one.

It is immoral if the "use" of sufferers is *beyond the desirable limits of use* for a noble purpose, which is touted to be benevolent. However, more and more "involvement" of sufferers in evaluating the ethic of "use" is not faced with any immorality. Is it really so? No perhaps, because beyond the *limits of "involvement" of patients* in ethical judgments of "use", something turns to be immoral. Here I have no business to go on evaluating the ethic of use of patients in medical education though there are a number of papers written on this matter. But many ethicists strongly argue that identification of "limits" or "desirable limits" is extremely important, which is possible if we keep in mind the points such as, rights to privacy and dignity of patients when it comes to frequent exposures or unnecessary exposures of patients, rights of patients in health care decision-making in the context of the enhancement of biological well-being, rights of patients in voluntary trials and tests in the context of advancement of physiological and diagnostic knowledge and right of patients to confidentiality in the context of disclosure of maladies for public safeguard. What interests me most in this regard is however the limits of "involvement" of patients in ethical and bioethical teaching to prospective or professional physicians and even nurses because some "ethics" is involved here as well. We should be extremely careful towards the right of the patients to participate in advancement of knowledge in the context of our greater urge to *disclose* their own medical preferences. It may be a little cunning act, well tuned though to bare open what a patient himself feels is ethically good and bad, right and wrong in medical decision-making and allotments because in that way we might pressurize the public psyche or the administrative hard nuts or even the close people of the patients to accept the truth that nothing is so evil if patient has chosen an evil deliberately thus clearing the practitioner of his obligations and duties. Truly, exploiting physically and mentally fatigued or nearly crunching patients by providing a questionnaire to fill up or to answer them orally or to respond to ethical debates so that people "involved" in ethical resolutions are helped by that, which becomes a part of teaching ethics and bioethics as well, stands a good case for ethical scrutiny. Hence, the ethic of over indulgence with the involvement of patients in medical ethics curriculum or medical decision-making about value-laden matters by means of "taxing" them even though those people may be very supportive and positive, is a great issue. Interesting is to notice that both patients and healthy people should contribute to some extent in this ethical debate of "using" patients in the name of "involving" them in ethical resolution through dialogues or corroboration of views. When in reality "involvement" becomes "using" is a matter of public scrutiny in our health care institutions lest at these places, ethics teaching has any role to play. This may be true to some extent when it comes to ethical involvement of members of a bereaved family whose near and dear ones are facing acute health crises, which also raises some ethical dilemma for the medical men. This shows that "public involvement" in resolution of ethical crises in medicine and in teaching curriculum is a delicate issue; it has its unique problems such as over-use, over-expectation and the cunning. Yet, every attempt at taking ethics to common people is fraught with unique problems, which have to be faced adequately.

Many people want to *support* this way of teaching ethics to medical men with other *methods*, known as the *narrative* and *the life-story methods*. These methods do not want to replace the earlier methods as I understand it but challenges the idea that if not imaginary situations or cases (as often we find in case of ethical issues in reproductive methodologies), are not of much educative value, we cannot deny some value of use of "narratives" from real-life situations in teaching ethics and bioethics to medical men. To this may be added another method, which is complementary to "narrative ethics" but different from it in many respects, that is the "life-story" or "life-history" method believed to contribute to teaching ethics. We have to decide whether or not both these methods can be really effective in teaching ethics to our medical men, when they are considered separately or in relation to what we have been thus far supporting, and to give it a name now, *corroborative ethical method*. The *narrative ethical method* is essentially *philosophical* in nature as different from the *life-story method* which is essentially *sociological*. We must say that the *corroborative method* is *philosophical as well as sociological* in nature. To call narrative method philosophical is to say that in the decision-making and resolution of medical dilemma, which we now recognize as one important component of growth of knowledge of ethics and medical ethics through systematic teaching, personal narratives of participants or contributors in the said process of resolution-decision are most important. However, mere narration of participants' experiences and encounters in resolution-decision is not of great importance, more value is given to the *ethical analysis* of the narration of experiences and encounters so that the gossip or the arm-chair effect of narration is overwhelmed by an intentional act of subjects to reveal the ethic of situations in which subjects were placed. This intends to achieve an understanding of the meaning of the situations in which the contributors were involved. Hence, the method calls for proper ethical evaluation of the social, cultural and personal situations in crises. Once medical men are involved in this process, they *learn* through doing something most required for them to do. We have been harping on at least two things covered by the method of corroboration. One is that ethical debates move with ethically framed questions, which is not structured by virtue of ethicists' wishes because framing those questions need a lot of inquiry into public and professional reactions initially. Second is that moving through ethical debates, evaluation of individuals' conception of ethically right, just, good and desirable about problems in consideration is possible because non-philosophers or philosophers either disagree or agree on ethical matters based on their *ethical evaluation* of what they have experienced and encountered which in turn they also narrate in the course of debates. Hence, corroborative method of learning ethics and medical ethics covers some important components of the narrative method. Nevertheless, it adds something more, for instance, being careful about *social-scientific vocation* in arranging ethical debates amounting to resolution-decision, the method, unlike the former one stresses on collection of moral opinion at the initial stages of "arranging debates" which comes to selection of most competent parties and framing most effective ethical questionnaire. This, I believe is the heart of any dialogue leading to resolution-decision and surely common sense feels its *non-narrative* nature because ethicists or any other party trying to scrutinize the moral opinions and depths of the participants to arrange a dialogue and to frame questions do not encourage narrations, neither evaluates them. But his questions leave room in a dialogue for the participants to disclose moral views freely through competent narratives and their inherent ethic.

However, the charge of the supporters of the *life-story or life-history* method such as Gillon and Tovery[3] against the narrative method is that an individual's or some individuals' evaluation of *personal experiences* as reflected in narratives is at best a restricted way to resolve moral crisis. In this sense, the method remains "individualistic", and as such having hardly any value in a 'group dynamics' where many people, the medical and the non-medical men, the philosophers and the non-philosophers, the patients and their parties or those related to them form a huge complex group, each having experiences, encounters, intentional processes to evaluate the ethic of their narrations collected in life but each agreeing as well as disagreeing on various ethical and non-ethical points. Hence, we come to a stream of sociological thought in which the inherent ethical tone could be easily noticed. Can we overlook this? Certainly not. Thus, we have the life-story method that cares for these huge complex groups' ethical concerns for resolution-decision of ethical impasse by transcending narrations and their evaluations. The point of departure being "individuality", in the life-story method, which is rather based on a more "general" outlook where *patterns of actions of people* find exposure in decision-making by virtue of cooperation of professionals and patients. It is a method of entering into social life and thereby enriching our knowledge of ethics. This method being sociological than philosophical relies heavily on collection of data based on study of cases. Here, the researcher is not essentially the one who collects ethical opinions of people rather collects empirical evidences in the form of "life-stories" which are *not literary* in origin rather objective ones, as testimonies to what ethical decision-making would amount to if these stories were to be counted as valuable resources, not for an individual but for a large collection of people around us. These stories, therefore, transcend both the peripheries of the individuals who collected or uttered them and of the relevance of these stories to the individual who collected or uttered them. The stories collected through a social scientific vocation are *general* in nature; they enable us to realize how in medical ethical problems life-stories become practically relevant not directly in resolution but to extend our knowledge about "patient worlds" so that proper evaluation of ethical crises is made possible. If we now consider the corroborative method, we find that it has distinct advantages over this method of collection of "patient stories". First is that being *philosophical and sociological* in nature, the corroborative method sidesteps the inherent problem of life-story method of being just sociological. It is not only important to "enter into the realms of patient worlds" rather important to evaluate the ethical relevance of the stories found in that world. Second, an evaluation of these stories as found in those worlds is possible not in isolation but in cooperation, when those not in the groups of data collection and story-suppliers also come together to evaluate the ethic of stories. This is further needed for able resolution and subsequent decision-making in case of value-laden medical issues because mere "knowledge of patient world" does not help us in real dynamics of ethical resolution, and if we wash our hands off such *practical enterprise*, the academic value of story-method does not take us too far. Ethics teaching and medical ethics teaching is a complex challenging affair, it demands that prospective and professional doctors grow their ethical knowledge not by listening and reading but by participating in an enterprise involving many parties including patients if needed, with a huge gamut of narratives and stories but all transcend those things to "enter into a cross-examination of views about what is desirable in order to get out of a practical impasse". No medical ethical teaching is complete without this participation with people as I believe. Corroborative method is thus an essential part of teaching ethics and medical ethics; when we come to these narratives and stories, we find a place for them as well, and they are not left out in dialogues. What both narratives and story-methods leave out is serious though, they try to remain in the shell of academic cover but do not come out of the comfort zone to face the music of ethical debate, and more seriously, do not consider "post-corroborative analysis" of the ethical views of the public that gives us gems of normative theories in action. Biomedical ethics is thus, as I understand, a dynamic affair – 'learning by doing'.

NOTES

1. Beauchamp, T.L. in the "Introduction" to *Contemporary Issues in Bioethics*, Wadsworth, Belmont, 1999, p. 26.
2. *Ibid*, pp. 26-27.
3. Readers may refer to R. Gillon's and Phillip Tovery's papers in the *Journal of Medical Ethics* published respectively in 1997 (23: 3-4) and 1998 (24: 176-181) for a good reading of narrative and life story methods of ethical resolution contributing to growth of knowledge of medical ethics.

Bibliography

Alderson, Priscila and Goodey, Christopher, "Doctors, Ethics and Special Education", *Journal of Medical Ethics*, BMJ Publishing Group, London, *24*: 1, 1998.

Areen, Judith *et al.* (eds.), *Law, Science and Medicine,* Foundation Press, NY, 1984.

Ayres, David Jr. *The Statesman,* Kolkata Edition, 5.1.02.

Bayer, Ronald, "AIDS Prevention – Sexual Ethics and Responsibility", T.L. Beauchamp *et al.* (eds.), *Contemporary Issues In Bioethics*, Wadsworth, Belmont, 1999.

Bayles, M.D. *Reproductive Ethics,* Prentice-Hall, Englewood eloffs, NJ, 1984.

Beauchamp, T.L. and Childress, J.F., "Rachels on Active and Passive Euthanasia", in T.L. Beauchamp *et al.* (eds.), *Contemporary Issues In Bioethics*, Wadsworth, Belmont, 1999.

Beauchamp, T.L. and Le Roy Walters (eds.), *Contemporary Issues In Bioethics*, Wadsworth, Belmont, 1999.

Benatar, Solomon R. "Imperialism, Research Ethics and Global Health", *Journal of Medical Ethics*, BMJ Publishing Group, London, *24*: 4, 1998.

Bindless, Linda, "The Use of Patients in Health Care Education: The Need for Ethical Justification", *Journal of Medical Ethics*, BMJ Publishing Group, London, *24*: 5, 1998.

Brock, Dan W., "Voluntary Active Euthanasia", in T.L. Beauchamp *et al.* (eds.), *Contemporary Issues In Bioethics*, Wadsworth, Belmont, 1999.

Brody, Baruch, "The Morality of Abortion", in T.L. Beauchamp *et al.* (eds.), *Contemporary Issues In Bioethics*, Wadsworth, Belmont, 1999.

Brody, Howard, *Ethical Discussions In Medicine*, Little Brown, Boston, 1976.

Buchnan, Allen E, "The Right to a Decent Minimum of Health Care", in T.L. Beauchamp *et al.* (eds.), *Contemporary Issues In Bioethics*, Wadsworth, Belmont, 1999.

Callahan, Daniel, *Abortion, Law, Choice and Morality*, Macmillan, NY, 1970.

Callahan, Daniel, "Cloning: Then and Now", in T.L. Beauchamp *et al.* (eds.), *Contemporary Issues In Bioethics*, Wadsworth, Belmont, 1999.

Cassell, Jackie, "Against Medical Ethics: Opening the Can of Worms", *Journal of Medical Ethics*, BMJ Publishing Group, London, *24*: 1, 1998.

Chadwick, Ruth, "Is Nursing Ethics Distinct from Medical Ethics?" in Edgar Morcher *et al.* (eds.), *Applied Ethics in a Troubled World*, Kluwer, The Netherlands, 1998.

Childress, James F., "Mandatory HIV Screening and Testing", in T.L. Beauchamp *et al.* (eds.), *Contemporary Issues In Bioethics*, Wadsworth, Belmont, 1999.

Cohen, Carl, "Do Animals Have Rights?" in T.L. Beauchamp *et al.* (eds.), *Contemporary Issues In Bioethics*, Wadsworth, Belmont, 1999.

Darr, A.S., "Editorial", *Journal of Medical Ethics*, BMJ Publishing Group, London, *24*: 6, 1998.

Dedek, John F., *Contemporary Medical Ethics*, Andrews and McMeel, Kansas, 1975.

De Marco, Joseph P. and Fox, R.M. (eds.), *New Directions in Ethics: The Challenge of Applied Ethics*, Routledge and Kegan Paul, NY.

Eaton, Stephanie, "The Subtle Politics of Organ Donation: A Proposal", *Journal of Medical Ethics*, BMJ Publishing Group, London, *24*: 3, 1998.

Emanuel, Ezekiel J. and Dubler Nancy Neveloff, "Preserving the Physician-Patient Relationship in the Era of Managed Health Care", in T.L. Beauchamp *et al.* (eds.), *Contemporary Issues In Bioethics*, Wadsworth, Belmont, 1999.

Engelhardt Jr., H.T., "Right to Health Care, Social Justice and Fairness", in T.L. Beauchamp *et al.* (eds.), *Contemporary Issues In Bioethics*, Wadsworth, Belmont, 1999.

Feinberg, Joel (eds.), *The Problem of Abortion*, Wadsworth, Belmont, 1984.

Feinberg, Joel, *The Moral Limits of Criminal Law*, O.U.P., NY, 1987.
Fletcher, Joseph, *Morals and Medicine*, Beacon Press, Boston, 1954.
Fletcher, Joseph, *Situation Ethics*, Westminster Press, Philadelphia, 1966.
Fletcher, Joseph, *The Ethics of Genetic Control: Ending Reproductive Roulette*, Promethnes Books, NY, 1972.
Gilligan, Carol, *In a Different Voice*, Harvard University Press, Cambridge, 1982
Gillon, R., "Eugenics, Contraception and Ethics", *Journal of Medical Ethics*, BMJ Publishing Group, London, *24*: 4, 1998.
Glover, J., *Causing Death and Saving Lives*, Penguin, Harmondsworth, 1987.
Glover, Nicola, "Community Care – Some Problems, Different Epithet?", *Journal of Medical Ethics*, BMJ Publishing Group, London, *24*: 5, 1998.
Gutman, Huck, "Biological Confidence Game", *The Statesman*, Kolkata, Edition, 10.9.2001.
Hamilton, Michael (ed.), *The New Genetics and the Future of Man*, William B. Erdmans, Michigan, 1972.
Harris, John, "Should We Attempt to Eradicate Disability?" in Edgar Morcher *et al.* (eds.), *Applied Ethics in a Troubled World*, Kluwer, The Netherlands, 1998.
Harrison, B. W., *Our Right to Choose: Toward a New Ethic of Abortion*, Beacon Press, Boston, 1983.
Holmes, S.J., *Life and Morals*, The McMillan Company, NY, 1948.
Hope, Tony, "Ethics and Law for Medical Students: The Core Curriculum", *Journal of Medical Ethics*, BMJ Publishing Group, London, *24*: 3, 1998.
Hope, Tony, "Medical Research Needs Lay Involvement", *Journal of Medical Ethics*, BMJ Publishing Group, London, *24*: 5, 1998.
Hughes, Jonathan, "Xenografting: Ethical Issues", *Journal of Medical Ethics*, BMJ Publishing Group, London, *24*: 1, 1998.
Kamm, F. M., "A Right to Choose Death?" in T.L. Beauchamp *et al.* (eds.), *Contemporary Issues In Bioethics*, Wadsworth, Belmont, 1999.
Kant, Immanuel, *The Groundwork of the Metaphysics of Morals*, (Trans.), H. J. Paton, B.I. Publications, Delhi, 1979.
Kass, Leon R., "Is There a Right to Die?" in T.L. Beauchamp *et al.* (eds.), *Contemporary Issues In Bioethics*, Wadsworth, Belmont, 1999.
Keown, John, "A Reply to McLachlan", *Journal of Medical Ethics*, BMJ Publishing Group, London, *24*: 4, 1998.

Kieffer, G. H., *Bioethics: A Text of Issues*, Addison Wesley, Massachusetts, 1979.

Kushe, Helga, "A Nursing Ethics of Care? Why Caring is not Enough?" Edgar Morcher *et al.* (ed.), *Applied Ethics in a Troubled World*, Kluwer, The Netherlands, 1998.

Kushe, Helga, "Euthanasia", Peter Singer (ed.), *A Companion to Ethics*, O.U.P., Oxford, 1991.

Locke, John, *Second Treatise of Government*, C. McPherson (ed.), Hackett, Indianapolis, 1980.

Macklin, Ruth, "Artificial Means of Reproduction and Our Understanding of the Family" in T.L. Beauchamp *et al.* (eds.), *Contemporary Issues In Bioethics*, Wadsworth, Belmont, 1999.

Mahowald, Mary B., "Biomedical Ethics: A Precocious Youth", in J.P. De Marco and R. M. Fox (eds.), *New Directions in Ethics: The Challenge of Applied Ethics*, Routledge and Kegan Paul, NY.

Marquis, Don, "Why Abortion is Immoral?" in T.L. Beauchamp *et al.* (eds.), *Contemporary Issues In Bioethics*, Wadsworth, Belmont, 1999.

McLachlan, Hugh V., "The Unpaid Donation of Blood and Altruism", *Journal of Medical Ethics*, BMJ Publishing Group, London, *24*: 4, 1998.

Morscher, Edgar, Neumaier, Otto and Simons, Peter (eds.), *Applied Ethics in a Troubled World*, Kluwer, The Netherlands, 1998.

Noddings, N. L., *Caring: A Feminist Approach to Ethic and Moral Education*, University of California Press, Berkeley, 1984.

Nozick, R., *Anarchy, State and Utopia*, Basic Book, NY, 1974.

Orentlicker, David, "Health Care Reform and The Patient – Physician Relationship" in T.L. Beauchamp *et al.* (eds.), *Contemporary Issues In Bioethics*, Wadsworth, Belmont, 1999.

Price, John, Price David, Williams Gail and Hoffenberg Raymond, "Teaching Medical Ethics: Changes in Medical Students Attitudes as They Progress Through a Medical Course", *Journal of Medical Ethics*, BMJ Publishing Group, London, *24*: 2, 1998.

Quill, Timothy E., "Death and Dignity: A Case of Individualised Decision Making", T.L. Beauchamp *et al.* (eds.), *Contemporary Issues In Bioethics*, Wadsworth, Belmont, 1999.

Rachels, James, "Active and Passive Euthanasia", T.L. Beauchamp *et al.* (eds.), *Contemporary Issues In Bioethics*, Wadsworth, Belmont, 1999.

Ramsey, Paul, *The Patient As a Person*, Yale University Press, New Haven, 1954.

Ramsey, Paul, *Fabricated Man: The Ethics of Genetic Control*, Yale University Press, New Haven, 1970.

Ramsey, Paul, *The Ethics of Fetal Research*, Yale University Press, New Haven, 1975.

Rawls, John, *A Theory of Good*, O.U.P., Oxford, 1972

Regan, Tom, *The Case of Animal Rights*, University of California Press, Berkeley, 1983.

Regan, Tom (ed.), *Matters of Life and Death*, Random House, NY, 1992.

Regan, Tom, "The Case Against Animal Research", T.L. Beauchamp *et al.* (eds.), *Contemporary Issues In Bioethics*, Wadsworth, Belmont, 1999.

Reich, Warren, *Encyclopaedia of Bioethics*, McMillan, NY, 1995.

Resnick, David B., "The Commodification of Human Reproductive Materials", *Journal of Medical Ethics*, BMJ Publishing Group, London, *24*: 6, 1998.

Robertson, John A., "IVF, Infertility and the Status of Embryos", T.L. Beauchamp *et al.* (eds.), *Contemporary Issues In Bioethics*, Wadsworth, Belmont, 1999.

Rothman, Barbara Katz, "Infertility as Disability", T.L. Beauchamp *et al.* (eds.), *Contemporary Issues In Bioethics*, Wadsworth, Belmont, 1999.

Ryan, C. J., "Pulling Up the Runaway: The Effect of New Evidence of Euthanasia's Slippery Slope", *Journal of Medical Ethics*, BMJ Publishing Group, London, *24*: 5, 1998.

Seedhouse, D.F., *Ethics: The Heart of Health Care*, John Willey, 1988.

Seedhouse, D.F., "Against Medical Ethics: A Philosopher's View", *Journal of Medical Ethics*, BMJ Publishing Group, London, *25*: 1, 1998.

Sherwin, Susan, *No Longer Patient: Feminist Ethics and Health Care*, Temple University Press, Philadelphia, 1992.

Sherwin, Susan, "Feminist Ethics In Vitro Fertilization", T.L. Beauchamp *et al.* (eds.), *Contemporary Issues In Bioethics*, Wadsworth, Belmont, 1999.

Silver, Lee M., "Cloning, Ethics and Religion", T.L. Beauchamp *et al.* (eds.), *Contemporary Issues In Bioethics*, Wadsworth, Belmont, 1999.

Singer, Peter, *Animal Liberation: A New Ethics for Our Treatment of Animals*, Avon Books, NY, 1975.

Singer, Peter, *The Expanding Circle*, O.U.P., Oxford, 1981.

Singer, Peter, *A Companion to Ethics*, O.U.P., Oxford, 1991.

Singer, Peter, *Practical Ethics*, Cambridge University Press, Cambridge, 1993.

Singer, Peter, "On Comparing the Value of Human and Non-Human Life", Edgar Morcher *et al.* (eds.), *Applied Ethics in a Troubled World*, Kluwer, The Netherlands, 1998.

Steinbeck, B. (eds.), *Killing and Letting Die*, Prentice-Hall, NJ, 1980

Sumner, L. W., *Abortion and Moral Theory*, Princeton University Press, Princeton, 1981.

Thieroux, Jacques P., *Ethics: Theory and Practice*, Glenco Publishing Co., California, 1980.

Thomasma, David C., "When Physicians Choose to Participate in the Death of Their Patients", T.L. Beauchamp *et al.* (eds.), *Contemporary Issues In Bioethics*, Wadsworth, Belmont, 1999.

Thomson, Judith Jarvis, "A Defence of Abortion", T.L. Beauchamp *et al.* (eds.), *Contemporary Issues In Bioethics*, Wadsworth, Belmont, 1999.

Tooley, M., *Abortion and Infanticide*, O.U.P., Oxford, 1983.

Tovey, Phillip, "Narrative Knowledge Development in Medical Ethics", *Journal of Medical Ethics*, BMJ Publishing Group, London, *24*: 3, 1998.

Veatch, Robert M., "Justice: The Basic Social Contract and Health Care", T.L. Beauchamp *et al.* (eds.), *Contemporary Issues In Bioethics*, Wadsworth, Belmont, 1999.

Velasquez, Manuel and Rostankowski, Cynthia (eds.), *Ethics: Theory and Practice*, Prentice-Hall, NJ.

Vlasak, Dr. Jerry, 'Report', *The Statesman*, Kolkata Edition, April, 1998.

Warren, Mary Anne, "Abortion", Peter Singer (ed.), *A Companion to Ethics*, O.U.P., Oxford, 1991.

Wilson, Edward, *Sociobiology: The New Synthesis*, Harvard University Press, Cambridge, Mass, 1975.

Wilson, Edward, *On Human Nature*, Harvard University Press, Cambridge, Mass, 1978.

Winston, Robert, "The Promise of Cloning for Human Medicine", *Journal of Medical Ethics*, BMJ Publishing Group, London, *31*: 4, 1997.

Index